VMS

VISUAL MNEMONICS FOR PATHOLOGY

LAURIE L. MARBAS
Texas Tech University Health Sciences Center
Class of 2003
School of Medicine
Lubbock, Texas

ERIN CASE
Texas Tech University Health Sciences Center
Class of 2003
School of Medicine
Lubbock, Texas

Blackwell
Publishing

© 2003 by Blackwell Science
a Blackwell Publishing company

Blackwell Publishing, Inc., 350 Main Street, Malden,
  Massachusetts 02148-5018, USA
Blackwell Science Ltd., Osney Mead, Oxford OX2 0EL, UK
Blackwell Science Asia Pty Ltd, 550 Swanston Street, Carlton,
  Victoria 3053, Australia
Blackwell Verlag GmbH, Kurfürstendamm 57, 10707 Berlin,
  Germany

02 03 04 05 5 4 3 2 1
ISBN: 0-632-04644-9

Library of Congress Cataloging-in-Publication Data

Marbas, Laurie L.
    Visual mnemonics for pathology / Laurie L. Marbas, Erin Case.
      p. ; cm. — (Visual mnemonics series)
Includes index.
    ISBN 0-632-04644-9
      1. Pathology—Study and teaching. 2. Pathology—Atlases.
3. Mnemonics.
    [DNLM: 1. Pathology—Terminology—English. 2. Association
    Learning—Terminology—English. QZ 15 M312v 2002] I. Case,
Erin. II.
Title. III. Series.
    RB123.5 .M37 2002
    616.07–dc21
2002004634

A catalogue record for this title is available from the British Library

Acquisitions: Beverly Copland
Development: Julia Casson
Production: Jennifer Kowalewski
Cover design: Meral Dabcovich, Visual Perspectives
Interior design: Shawn Girsberger
Typesetter: International Typesetting and Composition, in India
Printed and bound by Sheridon Books, in Michigan

For further information on Blackwell Publishing, visit our website:
www.blackwellscience.com

Notice: The indications and dosages of all drugs in this book have
been recommended in the medical literature and conform to the
practices of the general community. The medications described and
treatment prescriptions suggested do not necessarily have specific
approval by the Food and Drug Administration for use in the diseases and dosages for which they are recommended. The package
insert for each drug should be consulted for use and dosage as
approved by the FDA. Because standards for usage change, it is
advisable to keep abreast of revised recommendations, particularly
those concerning new drugs.

CONTENTS

PREFACE

Visual Mnemonics is a study tool that aids in quickly learning and memorizing material presented in Medical Pathology. Two significant features of *Visual Mnemonics* are the long-term retention of material and the increased rate of learning. This allows the student more time to study the fraction of material not covered in the *Visual Mnemonics* book.

These illustrations were created to assist in my own studying, because I was always short on time to efficiently memorize facts, and then I was frustrated because I couldn't remember them longer than the hour after the test. As a mom of 3 small children my time for studying is limited and must be high yield 100% of the time. These illustrations allowed me to do that and many classmates also. Several classmates stated to me that their grades improved 10 points from one exam to the next. Also, we all agree that the long-term retention is incredible compared to traditional study methods of memorizing from lists or note-cards.

I have attempted to combine as many pertinent facts and functions into the illustrations as possible. This book is not meant to be an end all to your studying but it certainly can provide an efficient and more stimulating method of studying the material that is contained in the illustrations.

Some tips on using the pictures: look at them after you have read your class notes, or gone to class, etc. Then you will know what material is not covered in this book, and what material is deemed important in your particular curriculum. Also, write on them, color them, redraw them, add your own drawings to them—the more the illustrations are manipulated the more information will be retained in long-term memory. Some students rewrite notes to study, etc.—write this information in the book. It will be concise and everything will be in one place for you.

ACKNOWLEDGMENTS

Throughout my medical education I have been blessed with many opportunities which I thank the Lord for everyday. A special thank you must go to my grandmother, Maxine Turner, for watching my three children while I attended my first two years of medical school and without her none of this would have been possible. My husband, Patrick Marbas, is also deserving of a tremendous debt of gratitude for making many sacrifices for me, including driving 100 miles one-way to work everyday, so that I could attend medical school. In addition, much love to my three beautiful children, Emily, Jonathan, and Gabriel, for playing quietly while I study and giving me hugs of encouragement when I needed it the most.

A special thank you to Erin Case for her friendship and dedication to our project during difficult and trying times.

Also, thank you to Dr. Susanne Graham for taking time out of her busy schedule to help us edit this project. I would also like to thank my mother, Patricia Lockridge, for her creative support throughout this project. Her encouragement has been invaluable and greatly appreciated.

Finally, a debt of gratitude to fellow classmates Joe Roman and Jan Seddighzadeh, for their unselfish sacrifice of exchanging third year schedules with us which alleviated many of our worries during the production of this book. Thank you.

— Laurie Marbas

I would love to thank my beautiful family for helping me, while putting up with me at the same time. My husband, Jay, has been a triumph of love and support while working on this book. I truly thank him for helping keep me sane. He also gives great back rubs. My sweet three-year-old daughter, Violet, who supports me with hugs, kisses, and happiness. A special thanks to my beautiful mom, Christine, for her love and all the babysitting. A thanks goes to my dad, Roger, for inspiring me to go into medicine. A world of thanks goes to my best friend ever, Laurie, for being the best listener and chauffeur. Thank you, Laurie, for giving me this great opportunity.

— Erin Case

DEDICATIONS

To Joe Roman and Jan Seddighzadeh for their friendship and support

To my sweet nephew Logan Joseph Robinette

And to my beautiful family Patrick, Emily, Jonathan, Gabriel, and Grams
Love,
Laurie

I dedicate this book to all the incredible women in my life, including my grandmother, Gango, my mom, Violet, Nanny, and Laurie. They are all great inspirations and I love them dearly.

A special dedication to my late father-in-law, Jerry, for treating me so kindly when I truly needed it.
Love,
Erin

CONSULTANT

Suzanne Graham, MD
Associate Professor of Pathology
Department of Pathology
Texas Tech Medical Center
Lubbock, TX

REVIEWERS

Andrew Louie
Class of 2004
George Washington University
Washington, DC

Arleigh Trainor
Class of 2003
University of North Dakota
Fargo, North Dakota

Hogan Shy
Class of 2003
University of California-Davis
Davis, California

Corinne LeVon Quinn
Class of 2003
MCP Hannemann
Philadelphia, Pennsylvania

1.
CARDIOVASCULAR

NOTES

HYPERTENSION

Factors increasing risk include

- diabetes
  - ⇒ DM on shirt
- genetics
  - ⇒ DNA molecule necklace
- smoking
  - ⇒ cigarette
- obesity
  - ⇒ large man
- increasing age
  - ⇒ walking cane
- blacks are at greater risk than whites

Can lead to

- cerebrovascular accidents
  - ⇒ rocket hitting brain
- heart failure
  - ⇒ tired heart
- aortic dissection
  - ⇒ aorta splitting in half
- renal failure
  - ⇒ tired kidney

Pathology

- atherosclerosis
- hyaline thickening
  - ⇒ hyena thickening

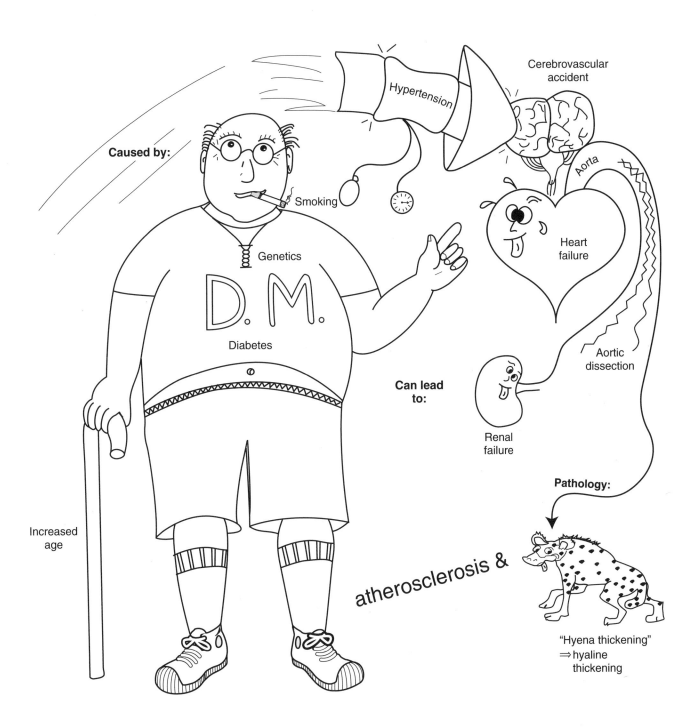

Caused by:

Hypertension

Cerebrovascular accident

Aorta

Smoking

Genetics

D. M.

Diabetes

Heart failure

Can lead to:

Renal failure

Aortic dissection

Increased age

Pathology:

atherosclerosis &

"Hyena thickening"
⇒ hyaline thickening

NOTES

PREECLAMPSIA-ECLAMPSIA

■ PREECLAMPSIA

Triad of proteinuria, hypertension, and edema
Presents around twentieth week of gestation
Occurs in 5% of pregnancies
Prelude to more life-threatening eclampsia

Clinical manifestations

- facial edema
- hypertension
  ⇒ blood pressure cuff
- abdominal pain
  ⇒ hand on abdomen
- extremity edema
  ⇒ swollen hand
- proteinuria
  ⇒ steak in urine
- hyperreflexia
  ⇒ reflex hammer hitting knee

Treatment

- salt restriction
  ⇒ salt shaker with line through it
- bed rest
- IV magnesium sulfate ($MgSO_4$)

■ ECLAMPSIA

⇒ E-clamp
- addition of seizures to preeclampsia triad
- left untreated it is usually fatal
- laboratory results include elevated liver enzymes, hemolytic anemia, and low platelets
- treatment is IV $MgSO_4$, but only cure is childbirth

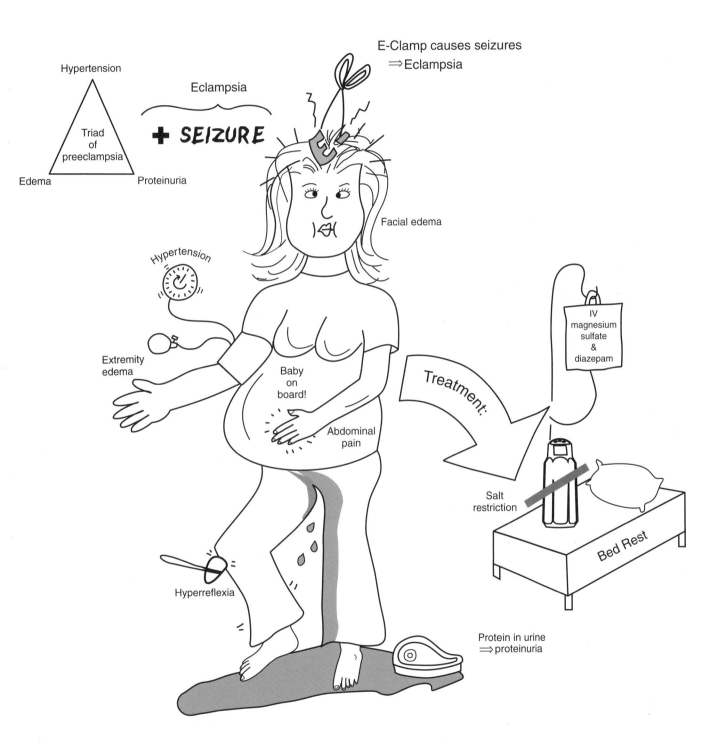

NOTES

Buerger's disease

⇒burger

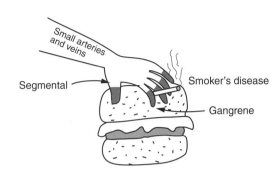

Small arteries and veins

Segmental

Smoker's disease

Gangrene

Temporal arteritis

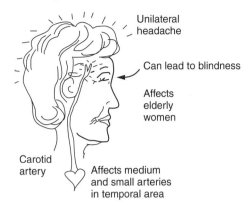

Unilateral headache

Can lead to blindness

Affects elderly women

Carotid artery

Affects medium and small arteries in temporal area

Takayasu's arteritis, aka Pulseless disease

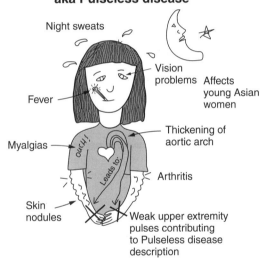

Night sweats

Vision problems

Affects young Asian women

Fever

Myalgias

Thickening of aortic arch

Arthritis

Ouch!!!

Leads to:

Skin nodules

Weak upper extremity pulses contributing to Pulseless disease description

Wegener's granulomatosis
⇒grand wagon

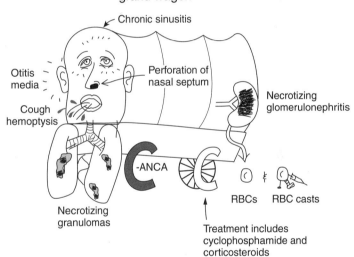

Chronic sinusitis

Otitis media

Perforation of nasal septum

Cough hemoptysis

Necrotizing glomerulonephritis

-ANCA

RBCs

RBC casts

Necrotizing granulomas

Treatment includes cyclophosphamide and corticosteroids

Polyarteritis nodosa

Hepatitis B association

Bee

It sure is getting hot!

Fever

Headache

Fever

Hypertension

Myocarditis & pericarditis

Cotton-wool spots

weight loss

PAN for P-ANCA

Kidney

Muscular

Affects small and medium muscular arteries, especially those of the kidney

ISCHEMIC HEART DISEASE

- ischemia is lack of oxygenated blood that results in insufficient oxygen and nutrients for the myocardium
- ischemia is caused by reduced coronary blood flow and increased myocardial demand
- four ischemic syndromes

1. **Angina pectoris**
   ⇒ angry pecs
   - stable (ST depressed) with coronary artery stenoses; exertion causes retrosternal chest pain
     ⇒ lowercase *s* and *t* in word *stable*
     ⇒ person pushing on word *stable*
   - Prinzmetal (ST elevated) with vasospasm
     ⇒ large *T* in word *Prinzmetal*
   - vasospasm
     ⇒ *T* having spasm
   - plaque disruption with mural thrombosis in unstable angina; chest pain gets worse
     ⇒ word *pain* under arrow pointing upward

2. **Myocardial infarction**
   ⇒ band-aid on heart

3. **Chronic ischemic heart disease**
   ⇒ days flipping by on calendar
   - seen in elderly patients with coronary atherosclerosis in whom congestive heart failure develops

4. **Sudden cardiac death**
   ⇒ tombstone with heart on it
   - death within 1 hour of symptoms
   - patients have atherosclerotic stenoses with acute disruption of plaque in coronary arteries that ultimately causes a fatal arrhythmia
     ⇒ lightning bolt hitting tombstone

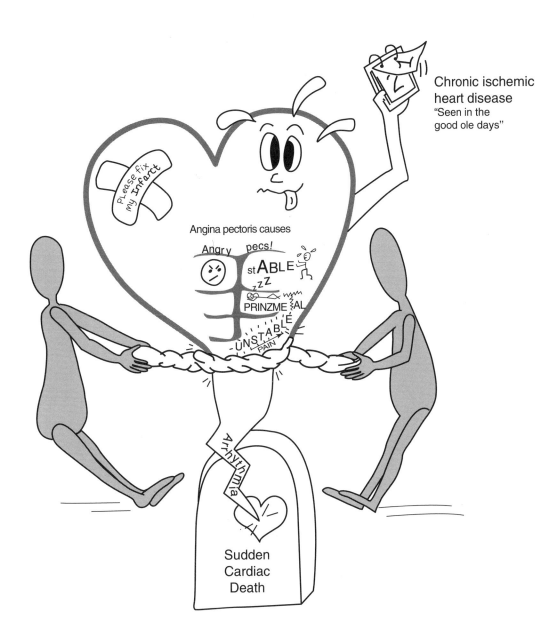

NOTES

BACTERIAL ENDOCARDITIS

⇒ in the card

Bacterial endocarditis can cause
- **MAJOR FeverS**, from **A cute fast *Aureus*** or **not so cute small vicious *viridans***
- **M**⇒murmur of new onset
- **A**⇒anemia
- **J**⇒Janeway lesions are small, painless, red-blue lesions that occur on the sole of the foot or the palm of the hand
- **O**⇒Osler nodes are red, raised, tender areas on the finger and toe pads due to infected emboli from the heart
- **R**⇒Roth spots are retinal white spots surrounded by areas of hemorrhage
- **S**⇒Splinter hemorrhages
- mitral valve is number one valve infected, and IV drug users often infect the tricuspid valve
  ⇒ "tricupid"
- acute endocarditis caused by *Staphylococcus aureus* quickly manifests on normal valves with large vegetations
  ⇒ **A** cute fast *Aureus*
- subacute endocarditis caused by *Streptococcus viridans* slowly manifests on previously damaged valves with small vegetations
  ⇒ not so cute small vicious *viridans*

Bacterial endocarditis can cause a
MAJOR FeverS, from **A cute fast** *aureus* **or not so cute** **small vicious** *viridans.*

Murmur
Anemia
Janeway lesions
Osler nodes
Roth spots
Fever
Splinter hemorrhages

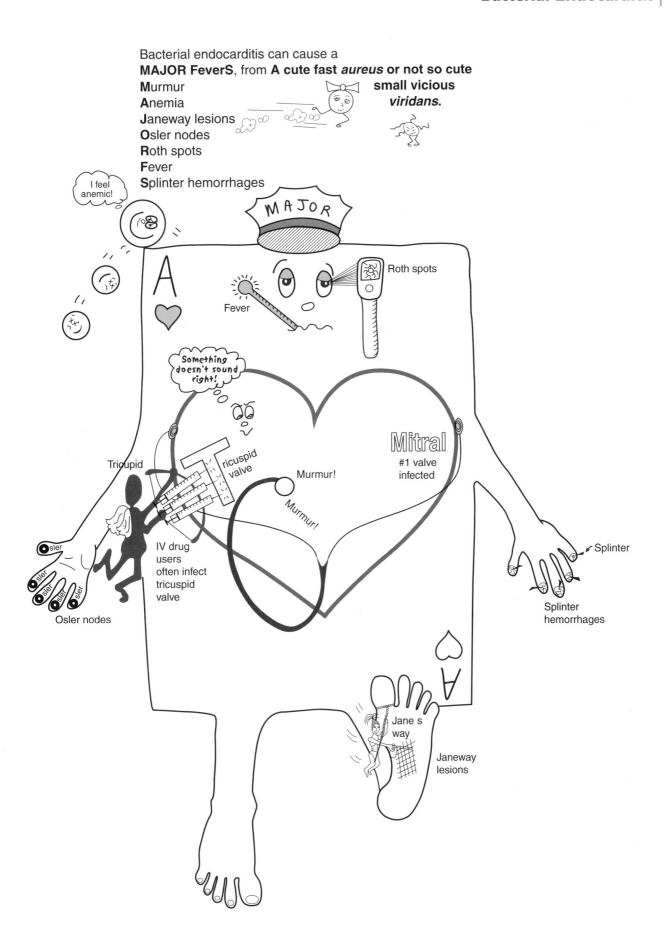

NOTES

CONGENITAL HEART DISEASE

- abnormalities of heart or great vessels
- cause of congenital malformations: genetic factors and environmental factors
- malformation categories: left-to-right shunt, right-to-left shunt, and obstruction
- right-to-left shunts: cyanosis occurs as a result of decreased pulmonary blood flow, and poorly oxygenated blood goes into the systemic circulation (cyanotic congenital heart disease); examples include tetralogy of Fallot, transposition of the great vessels, persistent truncus arteriosus, tricuspid atresia, and total anomalous pulmonary venous connection
- tetralogy of Fallot: four characteristics are ventricular septal defect (VSD), subpulmonary stenosis, aorta that overrides VSD, and right ventricular hypertrophy; degree of difficulty depends on severity of subpulmonary stenosis; heart is boot shaped
- transposition of great arteries: aorta arises from the right ventricle, and pulmonary artery originates from the left ventricle; incompatible with life unless some kind of shunt is present (e.g., VSD) that allows adequate mixing of the blood
- truncus arteriosus: failure of separation of aorta and pulmonary artery; single artery receives blood from both ventricles
- tricuspid atresia: complete occlusion of tricuspid valve; VSD is also present
- total anomalous pulmonary venous connection: no pulmonary veins directly join the left atrium; because a patent foramen ovale or an arterial septal defect (ASD) is always present, pulmonary venous blood enters the left atrium
- left-to-right shunt: examples include ASD, VSD, patent ductus arteriosus (PDA), and atrioventricular septal defects (AVSD)
- pulmonary blood flow is increased, and, therefore, cyanosis is not present; the increased pulmonary pressure results in pulmonary hypertension, which causes right ventricular hypertrophy and possibly failure; eventually, pulmonary pressure reaches systemic levels and the shunt is reversed to right-to-left, thereby sending unoxygenated blood into the systemic circulation (late cyanotic congenital heart disease or Eisenmenger's syndrome)
- ASD: abnormal opening in atrial septum (not a patent foramen ovale, which does not allow mixing of blood)
- VSD: most common congenital cardiac anomaly; Swiss-cheese septum (multiple VSDs in muscular septum)
- patent ductus arteriosus: persistence of connection between pulmonary artery and aorta; a machinery-like, continuous harsh murmur can be heard
- AVSD: superior and inferior endocardial cushions do not fuse adequately; associated with Down syndrome
- obstructive congenital anomalies
  - coarctation of aorta—narrowing of the aorta; females with Turner's syndrome have this disease; two forms are infantile (constriction proximal to PDA) and adult (distal to PDA); hypertension in upper extremities and weak pulse in lower, resulting in claudication; murmur is heard throughout systole; associated with rib notching
  - pulmonary stenosis and atresia: obstruction of pulmonary valve →right ventricular hypertrophy
  - aortic stenosis and atresia: can be valvular, subvalvular, and supravalvular (thickening of ascending aortic wall associated with Williams syndrome); can hear a systolic murmur and thrill

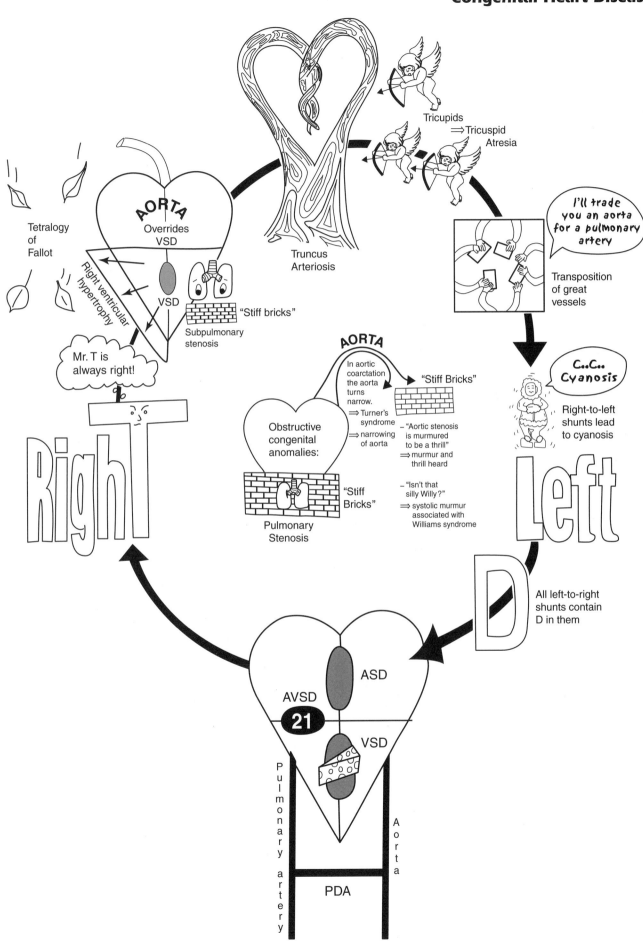

RHEUMATIC FEVER

- clinical findings: migratory polyarthritis of the large joints, carditis, subcutaneous nodules, erythema marginatum of the skin, and St. Vitus' dance or chorea
- diagnosis is made by the Jones criteria: evidence of group A streptococcal infection plus two major symptoms (listed above) or one major and two minor symptoms, including fever, arthralgia, or increased acute-phase reactants
- may cause rheumatic heart disease affecting the mitral valve
- most frequent cause of mitral stenosis
- "fish mouth" or "buttonhole" stenoses can occur when fibrous bridging across the valvular commissures occurs
- acute rheumatic fever occurs when antibodies against group A streptococci protein M cross-react with heart and joint tissue

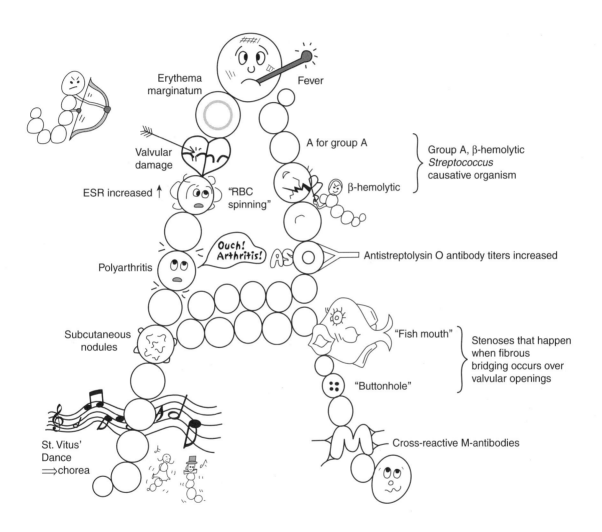

Erythema marginatum

Fever

A for group A

Group A, β-hemolytic *Streptococcus* causative organism

Valvular damage

ESR increased ↑

"RBC spinning"

β-hemolytic

Ouch! Arthritis!

Antistreptolysin O antibody titers increased

Polyarthritis

Subcutaneous nodules

"Fish mouth"

Stenoses that happen when fibrous bridging occurs over valvular openings

"Buttonhole"

St. Vitus' Dance ⟹chorea

Cross-reactive M-antibodies

NOTES

PERICARDITIS

- causes include
  - direct spread of pyogenic bacteria from lungs
  - tuberculosis (TB)
  - ischemic heart disease
  - uremia
  - rheumatoid arthritis (RA)
  - viruses
  - systemic lupus erythematosus (SLE)
- results in the following types of pericardial effusions
  - purulent
  - fibrinous
  - serous
  - serofibrinous
  - hemorrhagic which is associated with TB and malignancy
- leads to the following:
  - ST elevation on electrocardiogram (ECG)
  - pain
  - pulsus paradoxus
  - friction rub

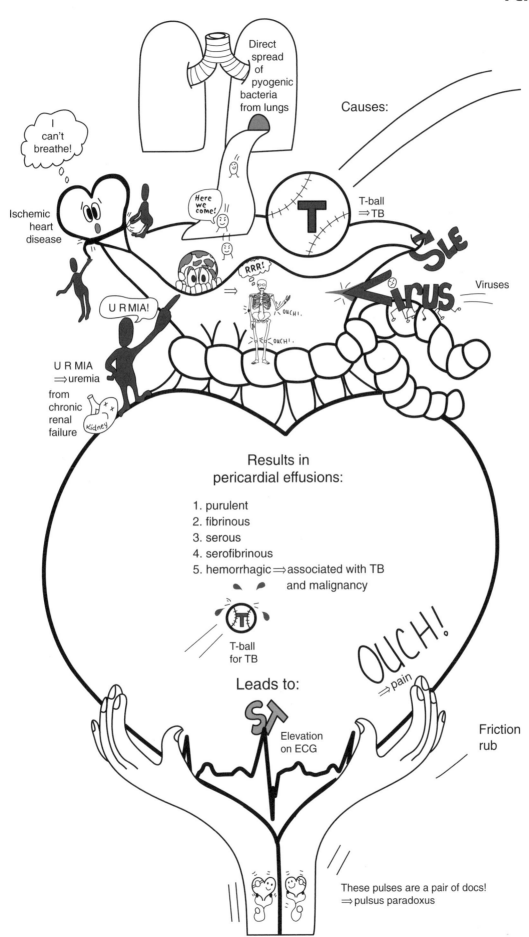

NOTES

MYOCARDIAL INFARCTION

- two types
  - transmural infarct: the entire thickness of vascular wall is affected
  - subendocardial infarct: inner one-third of myocardium is affected because it is most susceptible to ischemia; caused by diffuse coronary atherosclerosis or global borderline perfusion
- early damage (within 20–40 min) is reversible
- almost all transmural infarcts involve the left ventricle; the right ventricle is rarely infarcted alone
- reperfusion injury can occur with the generation of free oxygen radicals; necrosis with contraction bands occurs when irreversibly damaged myocytes are reperfused and the cell's membranes are exposed to a high plasma calcium concentration; myocytes reperfused may be stunned, which depresses function

Clinical Features

- patients present with rapid weak pulse, diaphoresis, dyspnea, or pulmonary edema; ECG changes include formation of Q waves
- laboratory tests measure intracellular macromolecule concentrations released from damaged myocytes (creatine kinase, of which creatine kinase muscle band [CKMB] is specific for the heart, and troponin I and troponin T)

Complications

- contractile dysfunction
- arrhythmias
- myocardial rupture: most commonly the ventricular free wall→leads to cardiac tamponade; second commonest is the ventricular septum→leads to left-to-right shunt; and third commonest is the papillary muscle→leads to mitral regurgitation; occurs 3–7 days after myocardial infarction (MI)
- pericarditis
- right ventricular infarction
- infarct extension or expansion
- mural thrombosis
- ventricular aneurysm
- papillary muscle dysfunction
- progressive heart failure

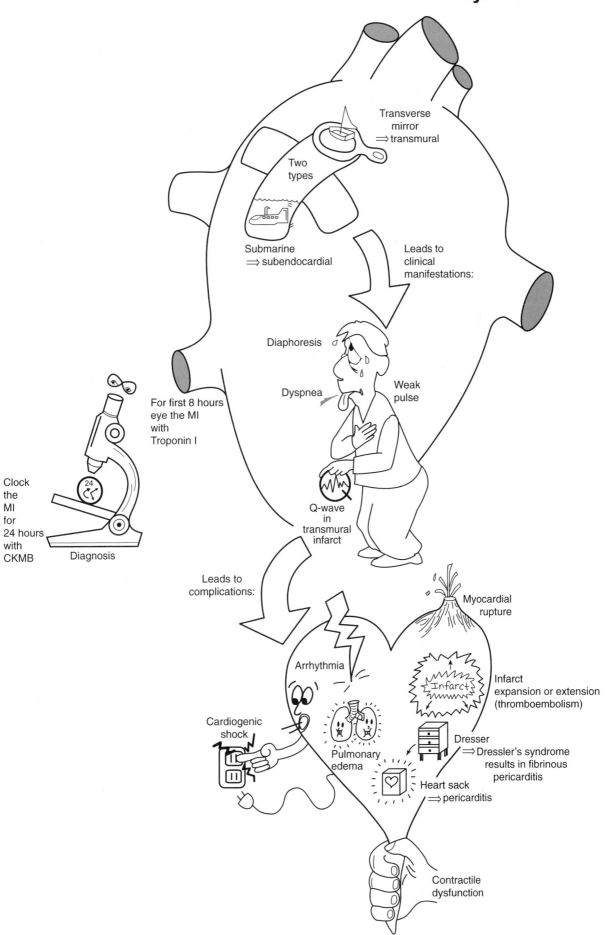

Transverse
mirror
⇒ transmural

Two
types

Submarine
⇒ subendocardial

Leads to
clinical
manifestations:

Diaphoresis

Dyspnea

Weak
pulse

For first 8 hours
eye the MI
with
Troponin I

Clock
the
MI
for
24 hours
with
CKMB

Diagnosis

Q-wave
in
transmural
infarct

Leads to
complications:

Myocardial
rupture

Arrhythmia

Infarct

Infarct
expansion or extension
(thromboembolism)

Cardiogenic
shock

Pulmonary
edema

Dresser
⇒ Dressler's syndrome
results in fibrinous
pericarditis

Heart sack
⇒ pericarditis

Contractile
dysfunction

NOTES

CARDIOMYOPATHIES

⇒ my **cardio** goes when studying **my path**!

- cardiomyopathy (heart muscle disease) is a heart disease that occurs from a primary problem within the myocardium
- the three types of cardiomyopathies are dilated (DCM), hypertrophic (HCM), and restrictive; the dilated form is commonest

Dilated Cardiomyopathy

- progressive cardiac hypertrophy, dilation, and contractile dysfunction; also known as *congestive cardiomyopathy*; has a hypocontractile heart and is a systolic disorder
- causes include myocarditis, alcohol, pregnancy, genetics, cocaine, doxorubicin, and beriberi
- the heart appears large and flaccid with all chambers dilated
- clinically, it presents with slowly progressive congestive heart failure and reduced ejection fraction, and death is caused by heart failure or arrhythmia

Hypertrophic Cardiomyopathy

- also known as idiopathic *hypertrophic subaortic stenosis* and *hypertrophic obstructive cardiomyopathy*
- distinguished by myocardial hypertrophy without dilation, abnormal diastolic filling, intermittent left ventricular outflow obstruction, and hypercontractility; diastolic disorder
- disproportionate thickening of the ventricular septum (asymmetric septal hypertrophy) is also present; cross-section reveals a compressed ventricle in a banana shape
- histologic features include myocyte hypertrophy and myofiber disarray
- disease can be of familial origin with autosomal dominant transmission; mutations occur in genes that encode sarcomeres
- clinically presents with reduced stroke volume from impaired diastolic filling of hypertrophied left ventricle, obstruction of left ventricular outflow, exertional dyspnea, severe systolic ejection murmur, and focal myocardial ischemia→causing angina
- one of the most common causes of sudden death in young athletes

Restrictive Cardiomyopathy

- primary decrease in ventricular compliance→impaired ventricular filling during diastole; systolic function is unaffected
- other restrictive diseases include endomyocardial fibrosis, Loeffler's endomyocarditis (with eosinophilia), and endocardial fibroelastosis (most common in first 2 yr of life)

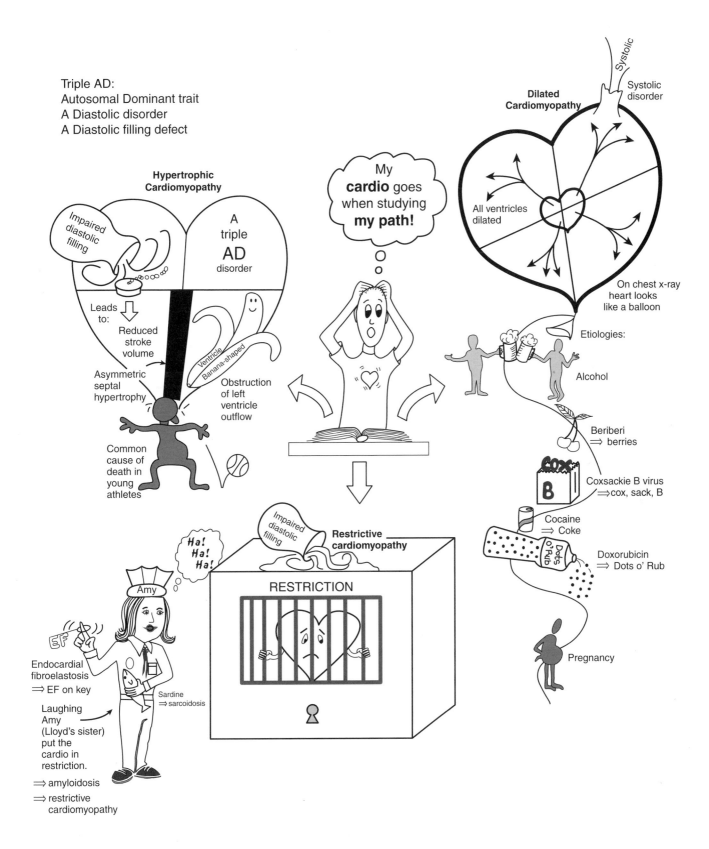

NOTES

CONGESTIVE HEART FAILURE

General

- defined as impaired cardiac function that leaves the heart unable to maintain a cardiac output capable of meeting the body's metabolic demands
- consequence of: systolic dysfunction→decreased myocardial contractile function or diastolic dysfunction→heart does not sufficiently relax during diastole for proper filling
- compensatory mechanisms: hypertrophy, ventricular dilation, blood volume expansion, and tachycardia

Causes of Right-Sided Heart Failure

- number one cause is left-sided heart failure
- pulmonary embolus

Leads to

- decreased forward venous flow
- liver congestion, also known as *nutmeg liver*
- peripheral edema
- central nervous system (CNS) and renal congestion

Causes of Left-Sided Heart Failure

- hypertension
- ischemic heart disease

Clinical Features

- paroxysmal nocturnal dyspnea (patient needs more pillows to sleep at night without dyspnea)
- orthopnea
- dyspnea on exertion
- other manifestations: histological→heart failure cells in lungs; decreased CNS perfusion; decreased renal perfusion→increased renin production and release

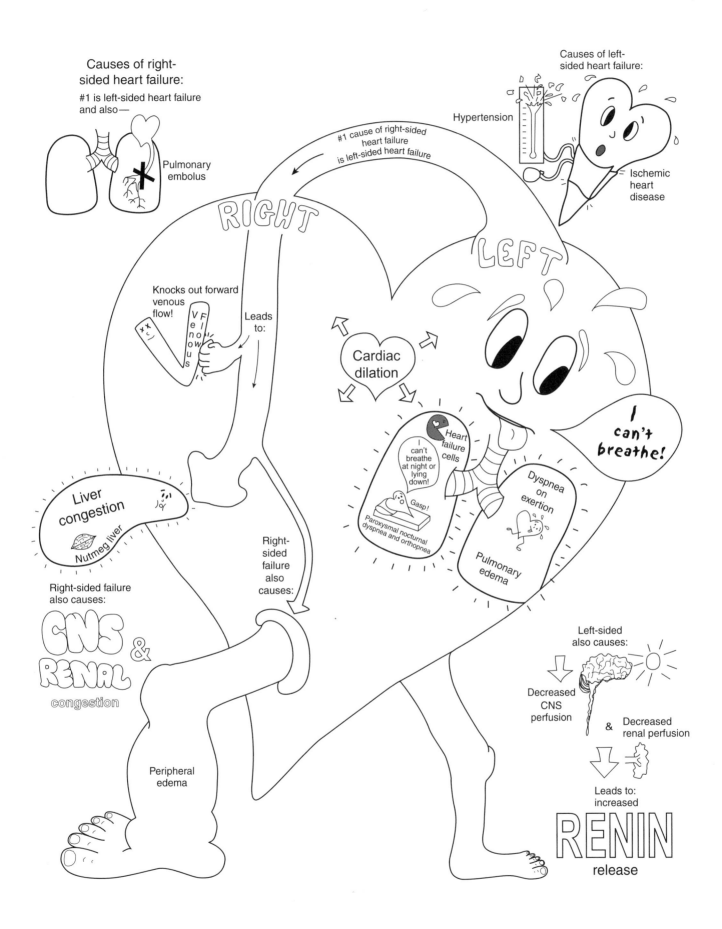

NOTES

NEOPLASTIC HEART DISEASE

- heart tumors are rare; metastatic heart tumors are more common
- primary tumors include myxomas, fibromas, lipomas, papillary fibroelastomas, rhabdomyomas, and angiosarcomas
- myxoma: most common tumor in adults; generally located in left atria; fossa ovalis is usual site of origin; occurrence is usually single; may exert wrecking ball effect due to mobility
- clinical presentation due to valvular ball→valve obstruction or embolization
- can be familial, in which case it is known as *Carney's syndrome*; autosomal dominant transmission
- lipoma: occurs in subendocardium, subepicardium, and within myocardium
- papillary fibroelastoma: usually located on valves; cluster of hairlike projections; similar to Lambl's excrescences
- rhabdomyoma: most common heart tumor in children; small, gray-white myocardial mass; contains spider cells; often associated with tuberous sclerosis
- sarcoma: angiosarcoma
- cardiac effects: metastases make it to the heart by retrograde lymphatic extension, hematogenous seeding, direct contiguous extension, or direct venous extension

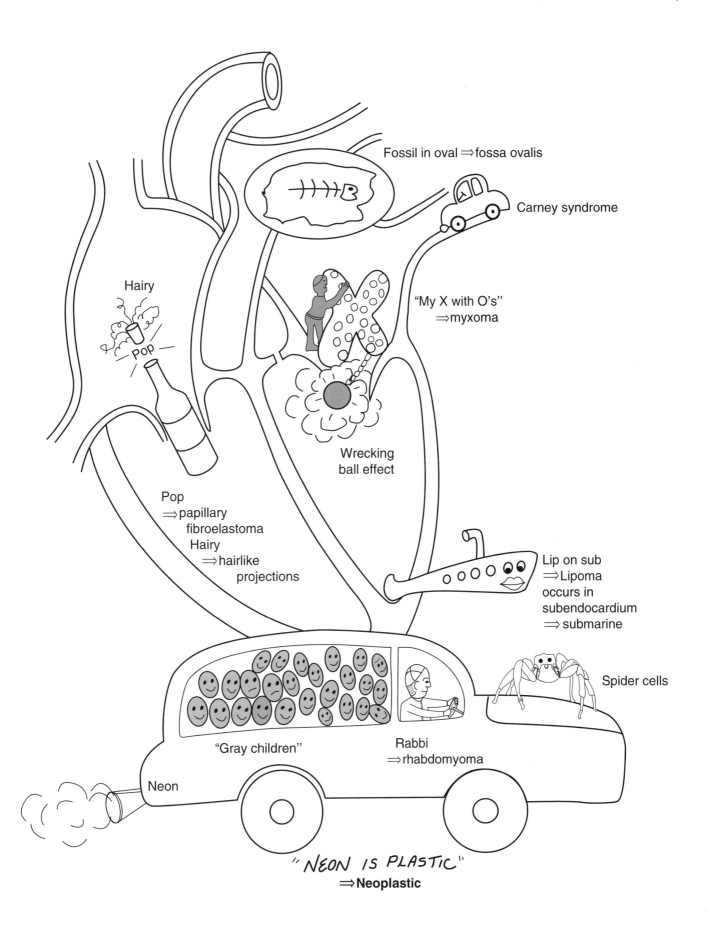

Fossil in oval ⇒ fossa ovalis

Carney syndrome

Hairy

Pop

"My X with O's"
⇒ myxoma

Wrecking
ball effect

Pop
⇒ papillary
fibroelastoma
Hairy
⇒ hairlike
projections

Lip on sub
⇒ Lipoma
occurs in
subendocardium
⇒ submarine

Spider cells

"Gray children"

Rabbi
⇒ rhabdomyoma

Neon

"NEON IS PLASTIC"
⇒ Neoplastic

NOTES

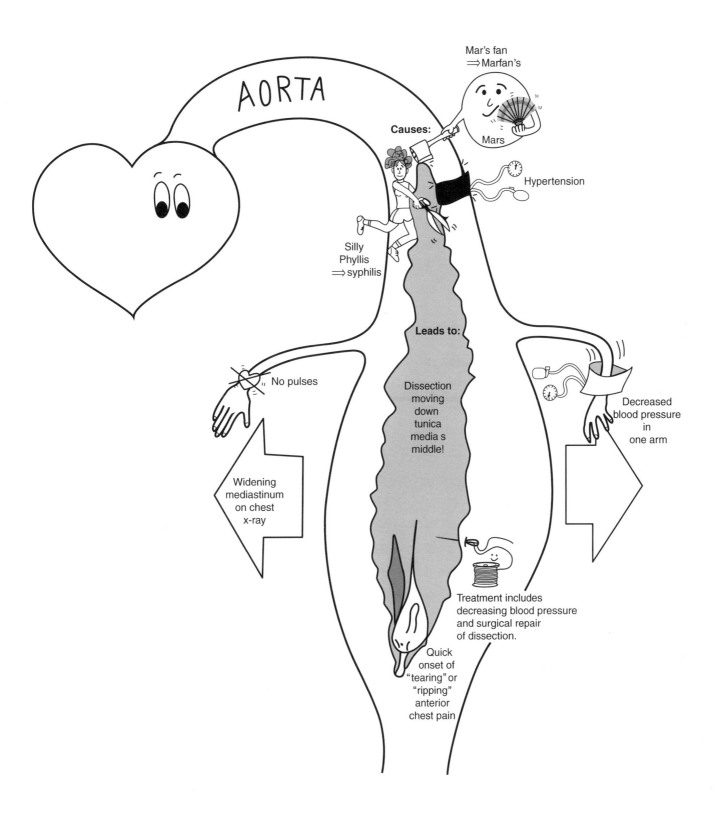

NOTES

MURMURS

In the…

Aortic Stenosis

⇒ frozen stiff
• systolic ejection murmur⇒silly
• crescendo-decrescendo⇒up and down

Aortic Regurgitation

⇒ whale regurgitates
• diastolic murmur⇒DIASTOLIC
• high-pitched blowing murmur⇒high-pressured blowing

Mitral Stenosis

⇒ mountain stiff
• left arterial (LA) pressure greater than left ventricular (LV) pressure
• murmur makes a "rumbling" noise⇒RUMBLE!

Mitral Prolapse

⇒ mountains overlap
• midsystolic click⇒silly click!

Mitral Regurgitation

⇒ wind regurgitated
• holosystolic⇒hole
• high-pitched blowing murmur⇒high-pitched wind

Patent Ductus Arteriosus (PDA)

⇒ shaped as a machine
• continuous machine-like murmur

Ventricular Septal Defect (VSD)

⇒ VSDVSDVSD
• holosystolic⇒whole silly VSD

Arctic
⟹ aortic

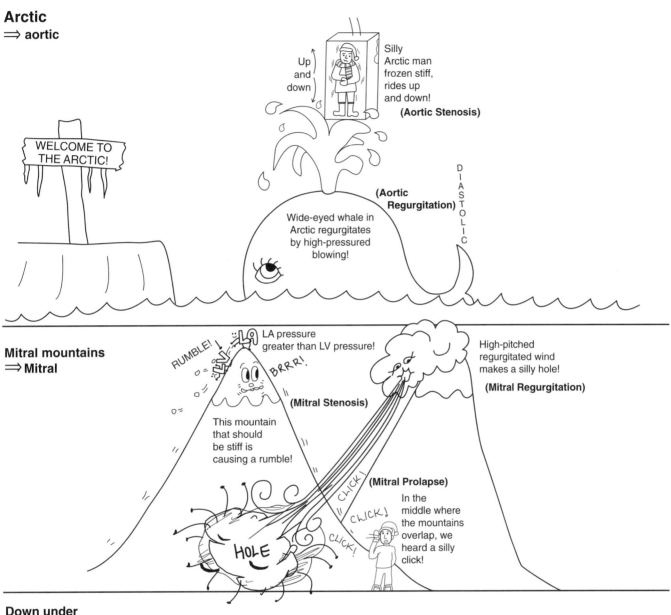

Up and down

Silly Arctic man frozen stiff, rides up and down!
(Aortic Stenosis)

(Aortic Regurgitation)

D I A S T O L I C

WELCOME TO THE ARCTIC!

Wide-eyed whale in Arctic regurgitates by high-pressured blowing!

Mitral mountains
⟹ Mitral

RUMBLE!

BRRR!

LA pressure greater than LV pressure!

High-pitched regurgitated wind makes a silly hole!
(Mitral Regurgitation)

(Mitral Stenosis)

This mountain that should be stiff is causing a rumble!

CLICK! CLICK! CLICK!

(Mitral Prolapse)

In the middle where the mountains overlap, we heard a silly click!

HOLE

Down under
⟹ D in PDA and VSD

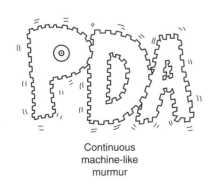

Continuous machine-like murmur

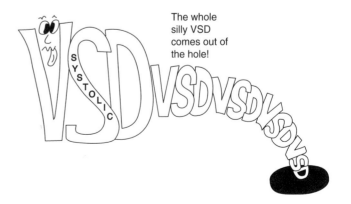

The whole silly VSD comes out of the hole!

S Y S T O L I C

2.
KIDNEY

NEPHROTIC SYNDROME DISEASES

Membranous Nephropathy

⇒ adult members only

- number one idiopathic nephrotic syndrome in adults; mean age 40 to 50; mostly men
- associated with human leukocyte antigen–DRw3; other associations include drugs (penicillamine, gold, catopril), infectious agents, systemic lupus erythematosus (SLE), malignancy with solid tumors (especially older patients)
- clinically presents with nephrotic syndrome, microscopic hematuria with no casts and no hypertension; renal function normal at presentation
- treat with prednisone or transplant (recurrence is not a problem)
- complications include renal vein thrombosis or superimposed anti–glomerular basement membrane (GBM) with crescent formation and clinical course like rapidly progressing glomerular nephritis (RPGN)
- subepithelial immune deposits (glomerular capillary wall destruction via complement [C5b-9])
- histologic findings include diffuse thickening of capillary walls (⇒ thick cap) without increase in cellularity; granular pattern of subepithelial immunoglobulin G and C3 deposits; electron micrograph (EM) shows subepithelial deposits with effacement of foot processes → spikelike extensions of BM→ thickening of BM→ with dissolution of deposits with clear area in BM

Minimal Change Disease

⇒ 1 cent is minimal change

- 75% of nephrotic syndromes in children; affects mostly 2- to 6-year-olds; most often male children
- one-third of patients have reduced glomerular filtration rate (GFR) or had preceding urinary tract infection
- renal function and blood pressure are normal
- nearly half spontaneously go into remission; treat with prednisone (⇒ Pred the cyclone) or alternatives cyclophosphamide or chlorambucil
- selective proteinuria; loss of negative charge on capillary wall; effacement of foot processes of epithelial cells⇒ fused feet
- associated with Hodgkin's lymphoma⇒ "hogs leavin' homa"

Focal Segmental Glomerular Sclerosis

⇒ arrow hitting focal point

- affects children and young adults
- causes include heroin-associated nephropathy (HAN)⇒HAN the hero,

human immunodeficiency virus–HIV malignant hypertension, and glomerulonephritis

- poor prognosis with nephrotic syndrome and hypertension
- treatment includes steroids, cyclophosphamide, chlorambucil, and transplants
- nonselective proteinuria, hematuria, sterile pyuria
- expansion of mesangial matrix causes capillary loop collapse
- PAS + intracapillary hyaline deposits; capillary tuft adheres to Bowman's capsule

Diabetic Nephropathy

⇒ diet of beets

- Kimmelsteil-Wilson lesions
- hyaline thickening of efferent and afferent arterioles

SLE

- renal involvement includes five patterns
- wire loop appearance
- granular subendothelial basement membrane deposits
- histologic findings include hematoxylin bodies and fingerprints

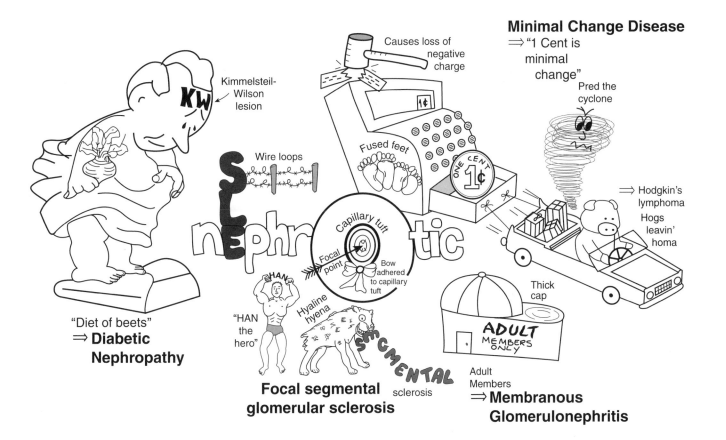

Kimmelsteil-Wilson lesion

KW

"Diet of beets"
⇒ **Diabetic Nephropathy**

Wire loops

Causes loss of negative charge

Fused feet

ONE CENT 1¢

Minimal Change Disease
⇒ "1 Cent is minimal change"

Pred the cyclone

⇒ Hodgkin's lymphoma

Hogs leavin' homa

Capillary tuft

Focal point

Bow adhered to capillary tuft

"HAN the hero"

HAN

Hyaline hyena

SEGMENTAL

sclerosis

Focal segmental glomerular sclerosis

Thick cap

ADULT MEMBERS ONLY

Adult Members
⇒ **Membranous Glomerulonephritis**

NOTES

NEPHROTIC SYNDROME

- NO hypercellularity, hematuria, or initial GFR reduction that is found in nephritic syndrome
- capillary wall permeability markedly increased
- initiating events include
  - primary kidney disease, minimal change disease (MCD), membranous nephropathy, membranoproliferative glomerulonephritis
  - malignancy (Hodgkin's lymphoma)
  - secondary kidney disease (diabetes mellitus, SLE, amyloidosis)
- insidious onset
  ⇒ sneaky fox
- proteinuria
  ⇒ hot dog links
- proteinuria leads to the following clinical findings:
  - hyperlipidemia
  - lipiduria
  - generalized edema
  - hypoalbuminemia
  - Maltese cross under polarized light
- complications
  - Fanconi's syndrome
    ⇒ fan
  - hypercoagulability
    ⇒ red blood cells sticking together as kidney's hair
  - protein malnutrition
    ⇒ kidney dropping meat (symbolizes protein)
  - acute renal failure
    ⇒ cross on kidney
  - reduced immunoglobulin G (IgG)
    ⇒ kidney stepping on IgG
  - vitamin D and trace mineral deficiencies
    ⇒ kidney stepping on vitamin D

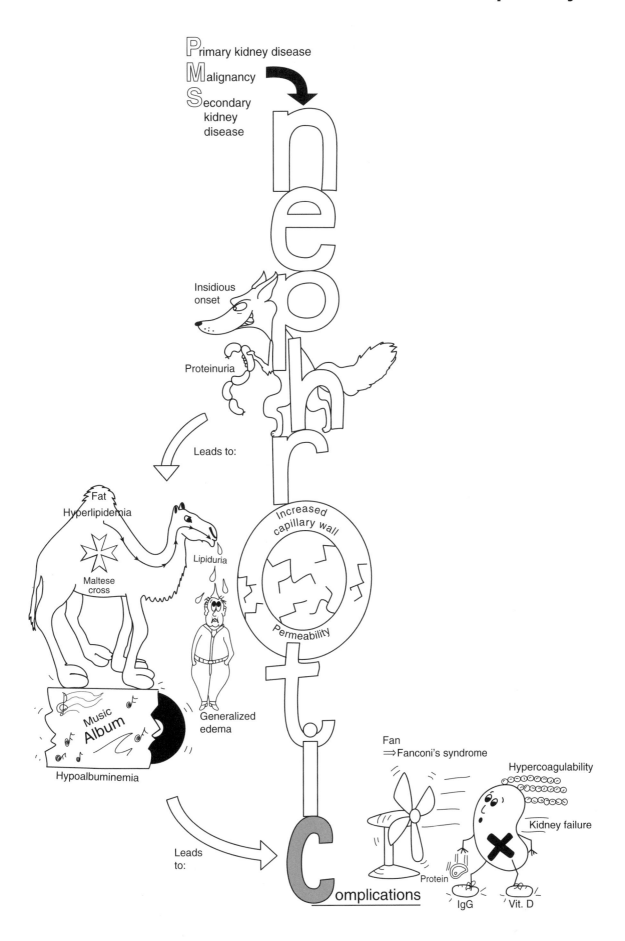

NOTES

NEPHRITIC SYNDROME DISEASES

Acute Poststreptococcal Glomerular Nephritis

⇒ a cute *Streptococcus*
- prototype of acute glomerulonephritis
- immune complex disease
- 2- to 12-year-olds most at risk
- boys are more often symptomatic
- treatment includes salt restriction
- self-limited course
- laboratory procedures include antistreptolysin O, streptoenzyme test, and reduced C3
- proliferative changes in capillary endothelial and mesangial cells→lead to narrowing of capillary loops
- subepithelial humps (granular deposits of IgG and C3) can be seen in EM; granular deposits can be seen with IF

IgA Nephropathy, Also Known As *Berger's Disease*

⇒ angel eating burger for Berger's disease
- immune complex disease
- glomerulonephritis most common
- 20- to 30-year-olds most afflicted; mostly men
- follows infection (upper respiratory tract, flu, gastrointestinal syndrome)
- macroscopic hematuria during or after infection (dysuria, loin, and flank pain associated); asymptomatic proteinuria; frequent recurrence
- histologic findings include focal segmental mesangial hypercellularity and granular IgA + C3 deposits in mesangium⇒messy angel

Goodpasture's Syndrome

⇒ pastor at podium
- affects young males
- patients with human leukocyte antigen DRw2 are at increased risk
- often preceded by flu or toxin inhalation
- 30% mortality due to pulmonary complications
- TRIAD: pulmonary hemorrhage, glomerulonephritis (hematuria, proteinuria, no hypertension or fluid retention), anti-GBM antibodies
- pathology includes antibody that binds GBM→fixes complement→recruits neutrophils and macrophages
- fibrin deposits in Bowman's space begin crescent formation
- histologic findings include early focal proliferative and necrotizing glomerulonephritis; later diffuse involvement and crescent formation; linear IgG deposition along capillary wall, and sometimes tubular BM

Crescentic (Moon) Glomerulonephritis Diseases (Rapidly Progressing Glomerulonephritis)

⇒ crescent moon; rapidly progressing glowing rulers
- rapid loss of renal function occurs with crescent formation (proliferation of Bowman's capsule's visceral layer with monocyte/macrophage migration) that eventually destroys Bowman's space

Membranoproliferative Glomerulonephritis

⇒ balloon lifts endothelium
- tram track appearance
- subendothelial humps or deposits of IgG and C3
- slow progression to renal failure

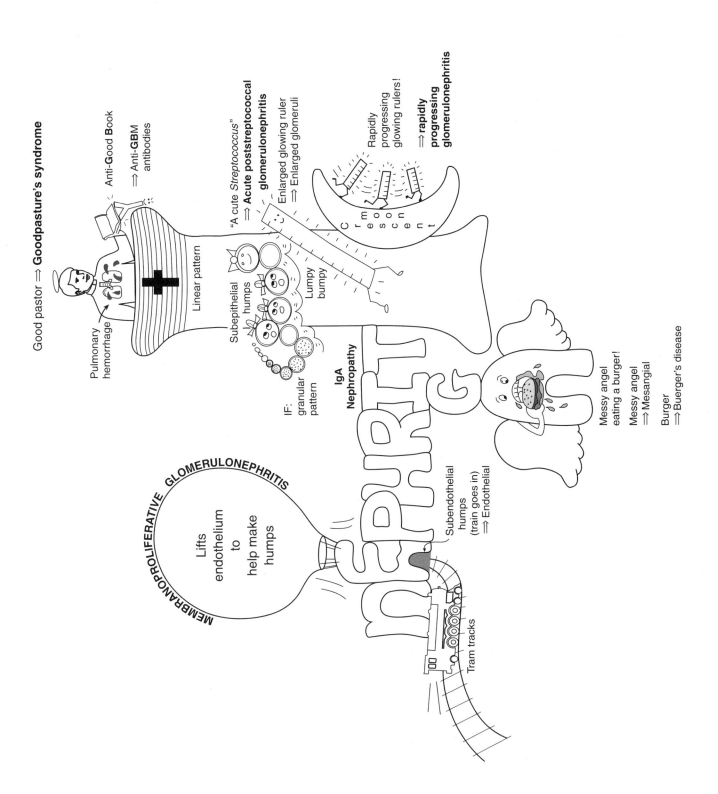

Good pastor ⇒ **Goodpasture's syndrome**

Anti-**Good Book**
⇒ Anti-**GBM** antibodies

Pulmonary hemorrhage

Linear pattern

"A cute *Streptococcus*"
⇒ **Acute poststreptococcal glomerulonephritis**

Enlarged glowing ruler
⇒ Enlarged glomeruli

Subepithelial humps

Lumpy bumpy

IF: granular pattern

Rapidly progressing glowing rulers!
⇒ **rapidly progressing glomerulonephritis**

Crescent

IgA Nephropathy

Messy angel eating a burger!

Messy angel ⇒ Mesangial

Burger ⇒ Buerger's disease

MEMBRANOPROLIFERATIVE GLOMERULONEPHRITIS

Lifts endothelium to help make humps

Subendothelial humps (train goes in) ⇒ Endothelial

Tram tracks

NEPHRITIC

NOTES

ACUTE NEPHRITIC SYNDROME

- abrupt onset of symptoms
  ⇒ man running fast
- glomerular hypercellularity
  ⇒ many glowing merry rulers!
- hematuria
  ⇒ blood drops falling into toilet
- proteinuria
  ⇒ hot dog links
- reduced GFR
  ⇒ arrow pointing down to show reduced GFR, urinary sodium, and RAAS→renin-angiotensin system
    ○ caused by compression of tufts by proliferating cells
    ○ thrombi in glomerular capillary
    ○ necrosis or obstruction by casts of tubules
- Na and water retention cause hypertension and edema
  ⇒ dam holding back sodium and water; hypertension ⇒ edematous man
    ○ also associated with gastrointestinal and central nervous system problems

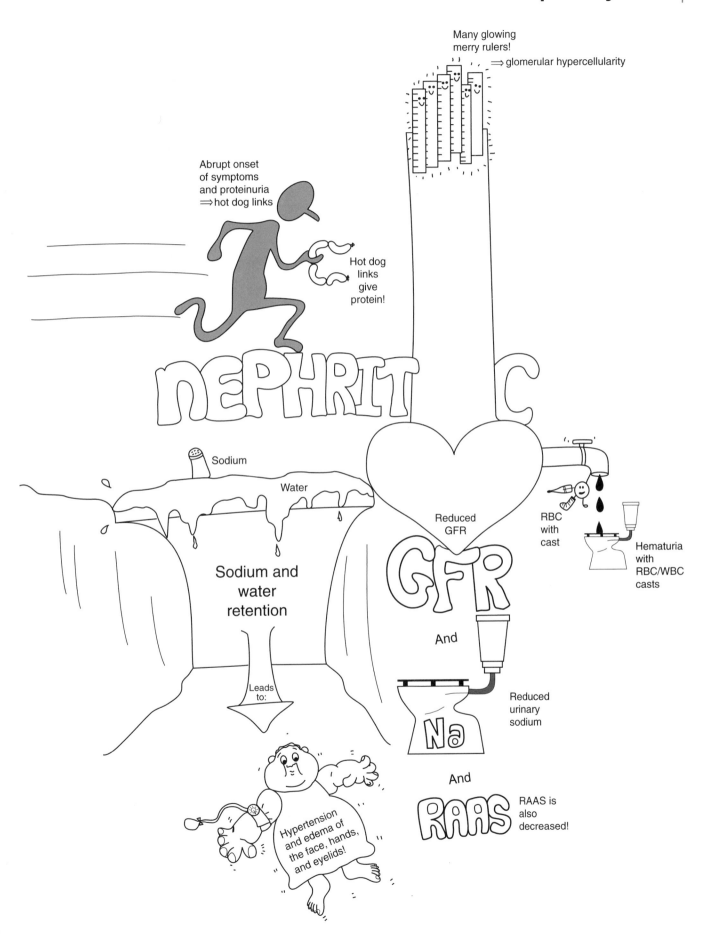

Many glowing
merry rulers!
⇒ glomerular hypercellularity

Abrupt onset
of symptoms
and proteinuria
⇒ hot dog links

Hot dog
links
give
protein!

Sodium

Water

Reduced
GFR

RBC
with
cast

Hematuria
with
RBC/WBC
casts

Sodium and
water
retention

And

Reduced
urinary
sodium

Leads
to:

Hypertension
and edema of
the face, hands,
and eyelids!

And

RAAS is
also
decreased!

NOTES

ANION GAP ACIDOSIS

- $Na - (Cl^- + HCO_3^-) = 8$ to 12 mEq/L
- Causes (MUDPILES)
    - **M:** methanol
        - $\Rightarrow$ me muddy
    - **U:** uremia
        - $\Rightarrow$ U aRE MIA!
    - **D:** diabetic ketoacidosis
        - $\Rightarrow$ diet of beets knocks me out!
    - **P:** phenformin or paraldehyde
        - $\Rightarrow$ fin form$\Rightarrow$pair of Als
    - **I:** isoniazid (INH) or iron tablets
        - $\Rightarrow$ INH$\Rightarrow$iron
    - **L:** lactic acid
        - $\Rightarrow$ lactic acid pouring on L
    - **E:** ethanol or ethylene glycol
        - $\Rightarrow$ beer on E's head$\Rightarrow$antifreeze
    - **S:** salicylates
        - $\Rightarrow$ aspirin bottle

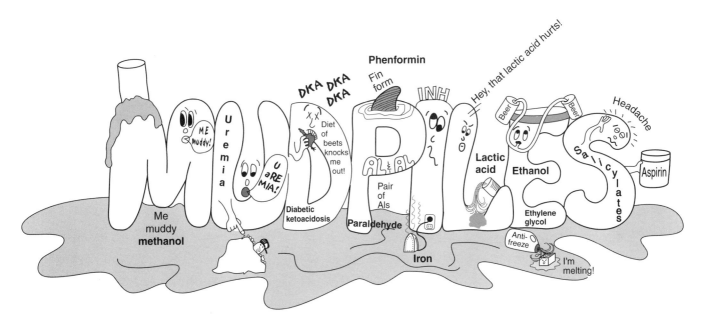

3.
LUNG

NOTES

CHRONIC BRONCHITIS "BLUE BLOATER"

- chronic obstructive lung disease
- ⇒ construction obstruction
- decreased FEV_1/FVC ratio
- results in air trapping and lung volume expansion
- ⇒ O_2 trapped and lung expanding
- caused by cigarette smoking
- infection maintains chronic bronchitis but does not initiate it
- hypertrophy of mucus-secreting glands leads to mucus plugs
- ⇒ electrical plug
- goblet cell proliferation in bronchi, bronchioles also leads to hypersecretion of mucus
- ⇒ many goblet glasses
- clinical manifestations
    - productive cough for more than 3 consecutive months in 2 years
    - wheezing
    - crackles
    - dyspnea on exertion
    - cyanosis; "blue bloater"
    - ⇒ sad (blue) bloated man
- can lead to
    - heart failure
    - ⇒ cracked heart
    - cor pulmonale
    - ⇒ apple core + pulmonary valve

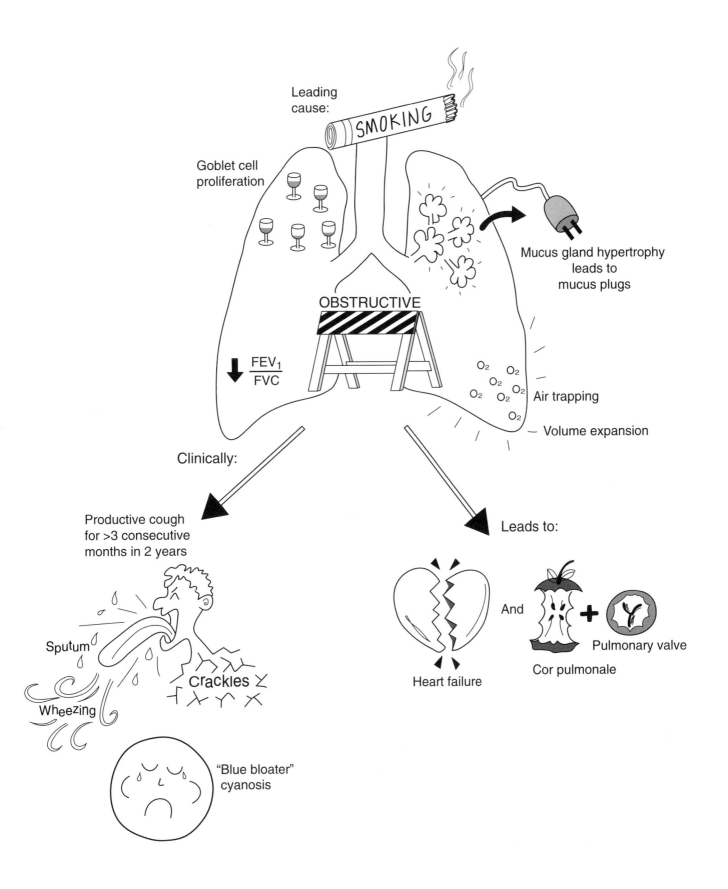

Leading cause: SMOKING

Goblet cell proliferation

Mucus gland hypertrophy leads to mucus plugs

OBSTRUCTIVE

↓ $\dfrac{FEV_1}{FVC}$

O₂ ... Air trapping

Volume expansion

Clinically:

Productive cough for >3 consecutive months in 2 years

Sputum

Wheezing

Crackles

"Blue bloater" cyanosis

Leads to:

Heart failure

And

Cor pulmonale

+ Pulmonary valve

NOTES

EMPHYSEMA "PINK PUFFER"

⇒ emphysema elephant; puffer fish
- destruction of alveolar walls
- enlargement of air spaces
- decreased recoil
⇒ coiled spring
- obstructive lung disease; decreased FEV_1/FVC ratio
- decreased inspiration-expiration (I/E) ratio
- types
  - centriacinar emphysema
  ⇒ "center of target on upper earlobe"
    - caused by smoking
    - affects upper lobes
    ⇒ "center of upper lobes"
    - occurs at the central or proximal parts of acini formed by respiratory bronchioles; distal alveoli are spared
  - panacinar emphysema
  ⇒ elephant on a pan
    - α_1-Antitrypsin deficiency
    ⇒ no tripping
      - results in an increase in elastase (protease); α_1-antitrypsin inhibits elastase
      - also associated with liver cirrhosis
    - most severe at lung bases of lower lobes
    ⇒ pan at elephant's base
    - acini are uniformly enlarged from respiratory bronchiole to terminal alveoli
  - paraseptal emphysema
  ⇒ parachute going up
    - distal acini involved; occurs in upper lobes
- clinical manifestations:
  - dyspnea
  - tachycardia
  ⇒ heart running fast
  - barrel chested
  - prolonged expiration; sit hunched over attempting to squeeze air out with expiration
  - blood gases usually normal due to overventilation

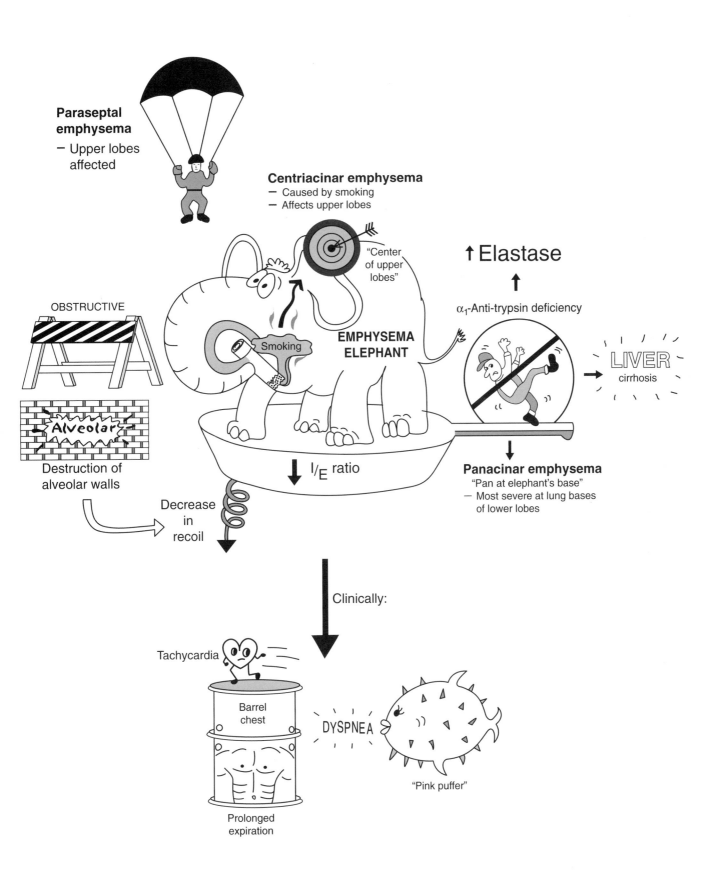

Paraseptal emphysema
- Upper lobes affected

Centriacinar emphysema
- Caused by smoking
- Affects upper lobes

"Center of upper lobes"

↑ Elastase

α_1-Anti-trypsin deficiency

OBSTRUCTIVE

Smoking

EMPHYSEMA ELEPHANT

LIVER cirrhosis

Alveolar

Destruction of alveolar walls

↓ I/E ratio

Panacinar emphysema
"Pan at elephant's base"
- Most severe at lung bases of lower lobes

Decrease in recoil

Clinically:

Tachycardia

Barrel chest

DYSPNEA

Prolonged expiration

"Pink puffer"

NOTES

ASTHMA

⇒ flames make ashes
- chronic inflammatory disorder
  ⇒ in flames
- reversible bronchoconstriction
- obstructive lung disease
  ⇒ construction obstruction
- decreased FEV_1/FVC ratio
- types
  - extrinsic: caused by type I hypersensitivity reaction from exposure to extrinsic allergen
    ⇒ exit sign
  - intrinsic: caused by nonimmune mechanism (viral upper respiratory tract infections [URIs], stress, aspirin)
    ⇒ enter sign
- clinically
  - cough, wheezing, dyspnea, tachypnea, hypoxemia
    ⇒ man coughing; hypoxemia⇒no O_2
  - decreased inspiration-expiration ratio
- morphology
  - Charcot-Leyden crystals: breakdown of eosinophils; red color
    ⇒ crystals
  - Curschmann's spirals: whorls of shed epithelium in mucus plugs
    ⇒ spirals
  - mucus plugs
    ⇒ electric plug
  - bronchial basement membrane thickening
  - hyperinflation of lungs

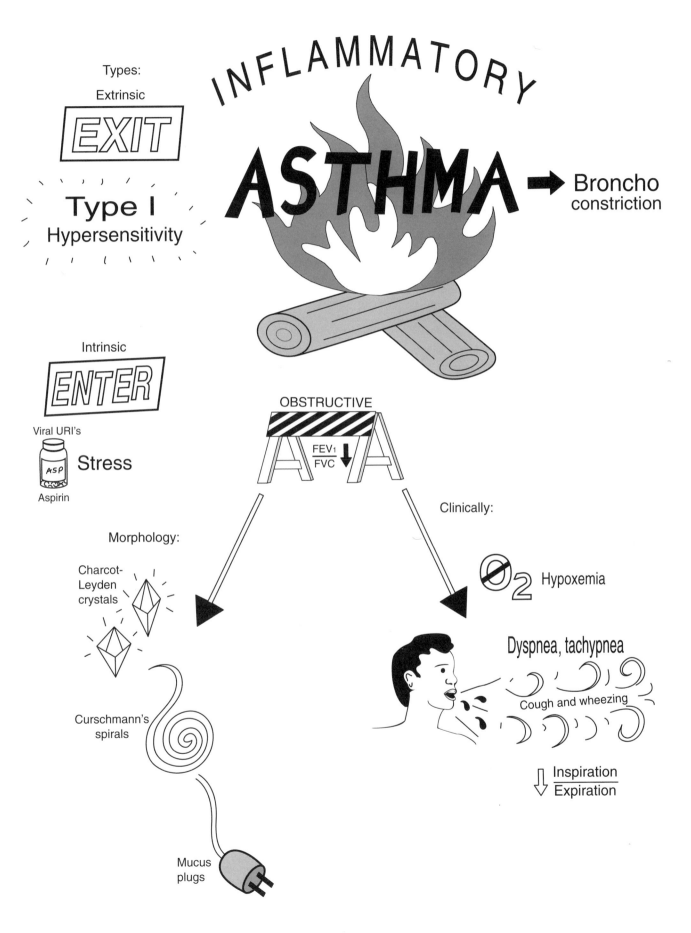

Types:

Extrinsic

EXIT

Type I
Hypersensitivity

INFLAMMATORY

ASTHMA → Broncho constriction

Intrinsic

ENTER

Viral URI's

ASP Stress

Aspirin

OBSTRUCTIVE

$\dfrac{FEV_1}{FVC}$ ↓

Clinically:

Morphology:

Charcot-Leyden crystals

Curschmann's spirals

Mucus plugs

O₂ Hypoxemia

Dyspnea, tachypnea

Cough and wheezing

$\dfrac{Inspiration}{Expiration}$

NOTES

BRONCHIECTASIS

⇒ bucking bronco
- chronic necrotizing infection in bronchi and bronchioles
- leads to permanent dilation of airways
- obstructive lung disease; decreased FEV_1/FVC
- caused by
    - cystic fibrosis (CF): autosomal recessive defect in CFTR gene results in defective chloride channel; thick mucus plugs in lung
    - Kartagener's syndrome: immotile cilia
    ⇒ car with tag
    - obstruction
    ⇒ construction obstruction
    - intralobar sequestration
- clinical manifestations
    - severe cough with foul-smelling purulent sputum
    - hemoptysis
    ⇒ bloody cough
    - fever
    ⇒ thermometer
    - orthopnea: breathing difficulty in any but an erect sitting or standing position
    ⇒ lying flat in bed causes breathing difficulty
    - cough usually occurs in the morning
    ⇒ sunshine

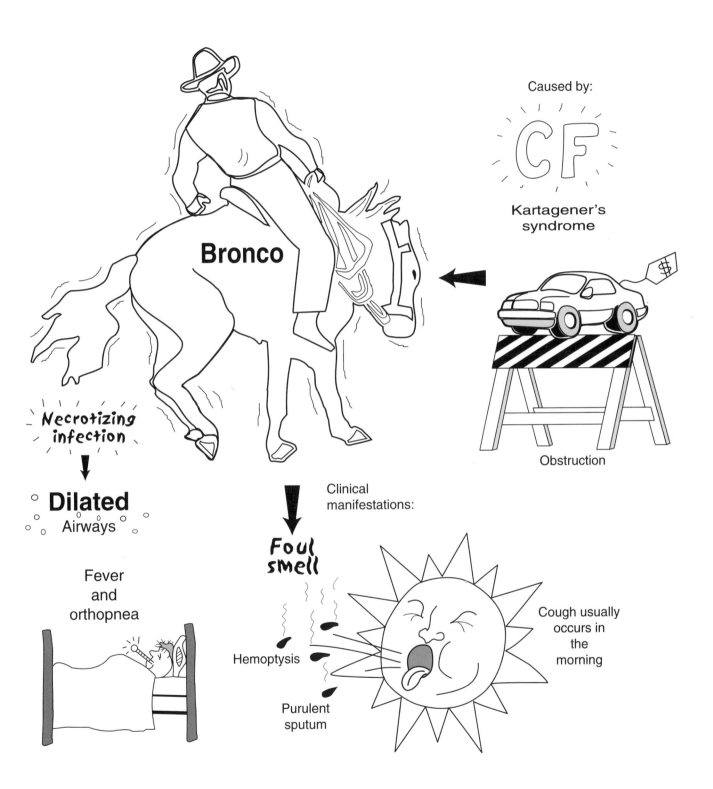

Bronco

Caused by:

CF

Kartagener's syndrome

Obstruction

Necrotizing infection

Dilated Airways

Fever and orthopnea

Clinical manifestations:

Foul smell

Hemoptysis

Purulent sputum

Cough usually occurs in the morning

NOTES

ARDS (ADULT RESPIRATORY DISTRESS SYNDROME)

- diffuse alveolar capillary damage increases permeability
- caused by
  - viral infections
  - ⇒ Viking virus
  - shock
  - O_2 toxicity
  - ⇒ oxygen tank
  - aspiration
- histologically
  - hyaline membranes
  - ⇒ hyena
  - type II epithelial cell proliferation: to regenerate alveolar lining
  - ⇒ many type IIs
- clinically
  - severe dyspnea and tachypnea
  - cyanosis
  - ⇒ ice cold man
  - arterial hypoxemia
  - ⇒ no oxygen
  - bilateral infiltrates
- lungs decrease in functional volume; ventilation-perfusion mismatching
- rapid onset of dangerous respiratory insufficiency, cyanosis, and hypoxemia leads to multiple system organ failure
- patients often die of bronchopneumonia
- ⇒ tombstone

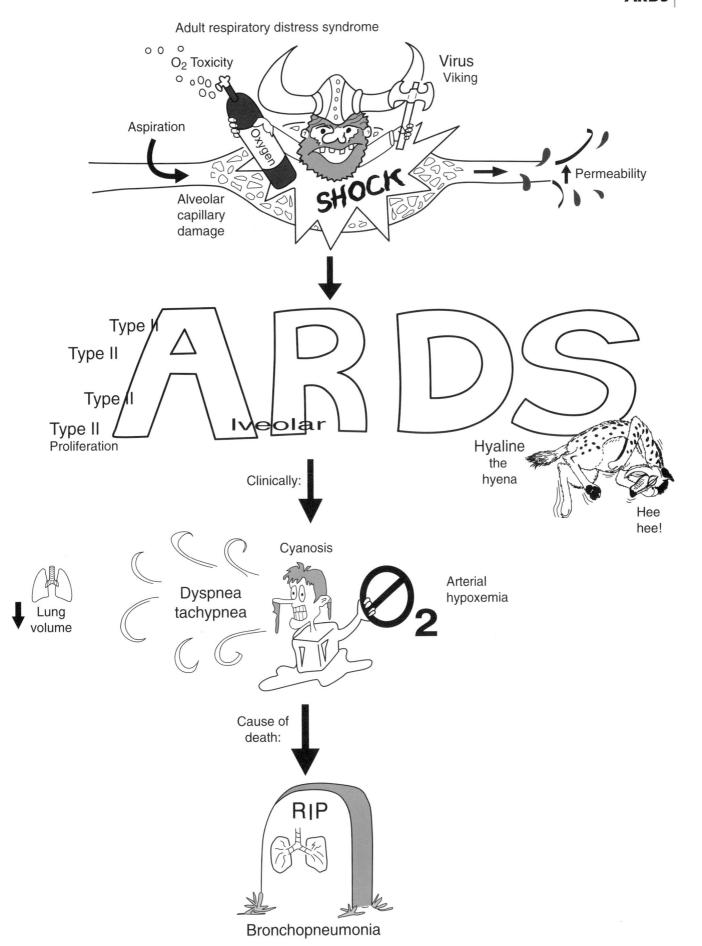

Adult respiratory distress syndrome

NOTES

SARCOIDOSIS

⇒ sardines
- systemic disease of unknown etiology characterized by noncaseating granulomas and an accumulation of T-lymphocytes and mononuclear phagocytes
- interstitial lung disease
- noncaseating granulomas
⇒ no case
- often seen in young black women
- microscopic features of granulomas
  - Schaumann bodies: laminated concretions of calcium and proteins
  ⇒ showman; hypercalcemia⇒milk
  - asteroid bodies: stellate inclusions enclosed in giant cells
  ⇒ asteroid and stars
- systemic manifestations
  - constitutional symptoms: fatigue, fever, weight loss, hemoptysis, and anorexia
  - fatigue⇒sleepy eyes; fever⇒ thermometer; hemoptysis⇒bloody cough
  - lung: hilar adenopathy, fibrosis; most commonly involved organ
  - eye: uveitis
  - skeletal: widening of bone shaft or new bone formation on outer surface; favors phalangeal bones of hands and feet
    ⇒ wide hand with bone
  - skin: erythema nodosum, subcutaneous nodules, plaques
  - liver: hepatomegaly
  - kidney: nephrolithiasis secondary to abnormal calcium metabolism

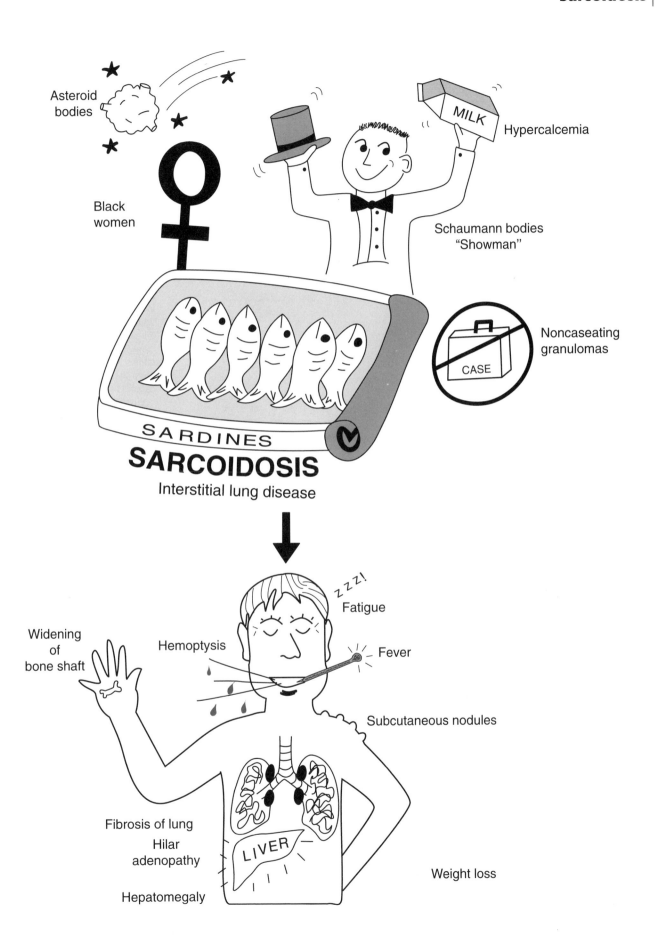

Asteroid bodies

Black women

Hypercalcemia

Schaumann bodies "Showman"

Noncaseating granulomas

CASE

SARDINES
SARCOIDOSIS
Interstitial lung disease

Widening of bone shaft

Hemoptysis

zzz! Fatigue

Fever

Subcutaneous nodules

Fibrosis of lung
Hilar adenopathy

LIVER

Hepatomegaly

Weight loss

NOTES

PNEUMOCONIOSES

- ⇒ pneumo cone
- reaction to mineral dust inhalation
- restrictive lung disease; FEV_1/FVC ratio greater than 80%
- interstitial fibrosis
- anthracosis (coal worker's lung)
- ⇒ ant as coal worker
  - caused by inhaled carbon particles engulfed by alveolar macrophages
  - accumulates along lymphatics
  - located in upper lobes
- silicosis
- ⇒ silly clown
  - caused by inhaled silica
  - most common occupational disease in the world
  - ⇒ "#1"
  - occurs in sand blasters, mine workers, and glass cutters
  - ⇒ sand castle, bomb in sand
  - increased susceptibility to tuberculosis
  - ⇒ T-ball
  - blackened nodules in upper lobes
- asbestosis
- ⇒ ribbon for the best O's
  - caused by inhaled asbestos fibers
  - occurs in plumbers and shipbuilders
  - ⇒ plunger
  - increased risk of mesothelioma and bronchogencic carcinoma
  - ⇒ messy can of CANCER
  - smoking further increases the risk of cancer
  - ferruginous bodies: asbestos fibers coated with hemosiderin
  - ⇒ furry rug and iron
  - may have calcified pleural plaques
  - irregular linear densities in lower lobes on x-ray

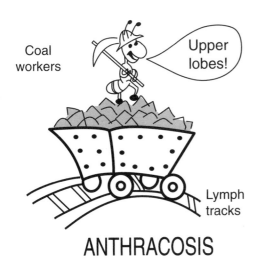

Coal workers

Upper lobes!

Lymph tracks

ANTHRACOSIS

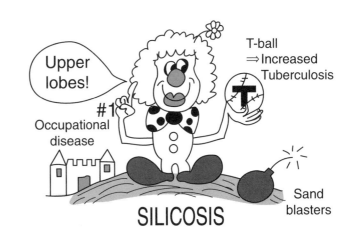

Upper lobes!

#1 Occupational disease

T-ball ⇒ Increased Tuberculosis

Sand blasters

SILICOSIS

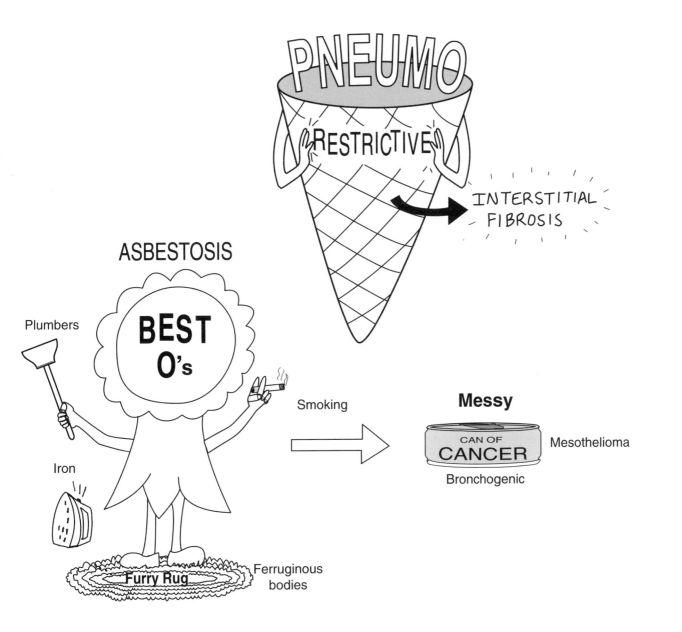

PNEUMO

RESTRICTIVE

INTERSTITIAL FIBROSIS

ASBESTOSIS

BEST O's

Plumbers

Iron

Furry Rug

Ferruginous bodies

Smoking

Messy

CAN OF CANCER

Mesothelioma

Bronchogenic

NOTES

LUNG CANCER
⇒ can of CANCER

Central Arising Tumors

- squamous cell carcinoma
    - ⇒ scale
    - associated with smoking
    - parathyroid hormone (PTH)-like production leads to hypercalcemia
        - ⇒ increase in Ca^{2+}
    - formation of keratin pearls and intracellular bridges
        - ⇒ carrots and pearls
- small cell carcinoma
    - ⇒ small jail cell
    - associated with smoking
    - ectopic antidiuretic hormone (ADH) and adrenocorticotropic hormone (ACTH) production
    - Oat cells present
    - forms clusters of basophilic cells
        - ⇒ grape clusters
    - responds well to chemotherapy

Peripheral Arising Tumors

- adenocarcinoma:
    - ⇒ "add in no carcinoma!"
    - most common in women and nonsmokers
    - mucin production
- large cell carcinoma
    - undifferentiated
    - clear cells

Clinical Manifestations

- cough and hemoptysis
    - ⇒ bloody cough
- weight loss
- bronchial obstruction
- coin lesion on x-ray
    - ⇒ 1 cent coin

Complications

- superior vena cava (SVC) syndrome: obstruction of SVC leads to facial swelling, vein dilation, and cyanosis
    - ⇒ cave with crown
- Pancoast's tumor: tumor in apex of lung that compresses cervical sympathetics, leading to Horner's syndrome
    - ⇒ pan
- Horner's syndrome: ptosis, miosis, and anhydrosis
    - ⇒ horns on cave
- pleural effusions
- paraneoplastic syndromes (PTH, ADH, ACTH)
- hoarseness from recurrent laryngeal nerve involvement

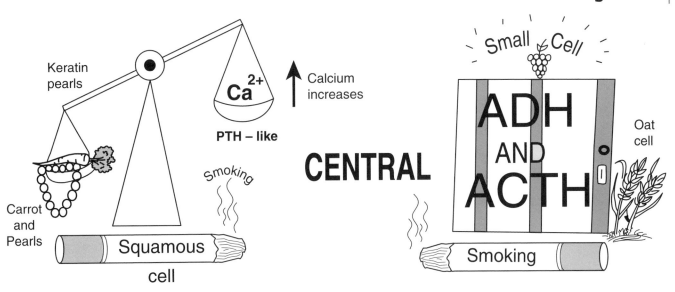

Keratin pearls

Ca^{2+} ↑ Calcium increases

PTH – like

Carrot and Pearls

Smoking

Squamous cell

Small Cell

CENTRAL

ADH AND ACTH

Oat cell

Smoking

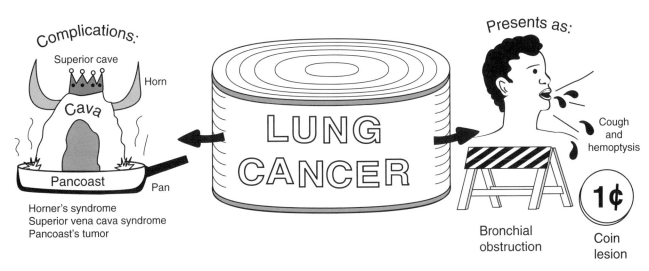

Complications:

Superior cave

Horn

Cava

Pancoast

Pan

Horner's syndrome
Superior vena cava syndrome
Pancoast's tumor

LUNG CANCER

Presents as:

Cough and hemoptysis

Bronchial obstruction

1¢

Coin lesion

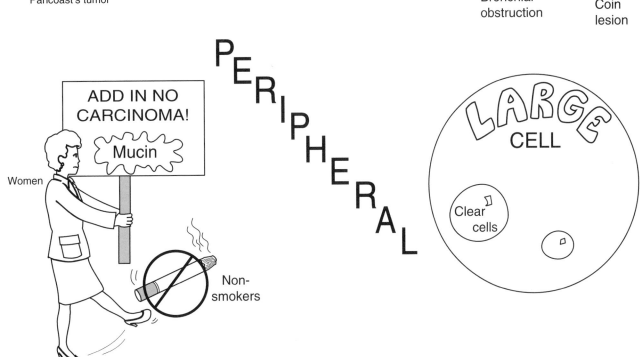

P E R I P H E R A L

ADD IN NO CARCINOMA!

Mucin

Women

Non-smokers

Adenocarcinoma

LARGE CELL

Clear cells

NOTES

LUNG INFECTIONS

Tuberculosis: Infection With *Mycobacterium tuberculosis*

⇒ T-ball
- primary: Ghon complexes present, usually in lower lobes
  ⇒ T-ball is Gone (Ghon); primary is one finger
- bloodborne spread when activated
- secondary: reactivation results in tubercle formation, cavitary lesions, and caseous necrosis; located in apex of lungs
  ⇒ apex of mountains, case for caseous

Mycoplasma*: Infection with *Mycoplasma pneumoniae

⇒ my cop and plasma
- cause of atypical "walking" pneumonia
- causes interstitial pneumonia
- presents as dry cough with no alveolar exudates
- hyaline in alveolar walls
- cold agglutinin in serum
  ⇒ cold glue

Abscess

- caused by aspiration
- more common on the right lung
  ⇒ air-fluid level in right lung
- air-fluid level present
- gangrene can occur with continued infection

Pneumonia

- bronchopneumonia: infiltrates in bronchioles and adjacent alveoli
  ⇒ bronco with patches
  ○ patchy distribution
  ○ caused by *Haemophilus* flu, *Staphylococcus aureus*, and *Staphylococcus pyogenes*
    ⇒ H with wings flew; cocci in shape of staff (*Staph*)
- lobar pneumonia: exudates in alveoli
  ⇒ earlobe
  ○ forms a consolidation
  ○ caused by: *Streptococcus pneumoniae*
- interstitial pneumonia: inflammation of interstitial areas
  ⇒ viruses and myco enter and diffuse
  ○ diffuse distribution
  ○ caused by: respiratory syncytial virus (RSV), adenovirus, and *Mycoplasma*

1° TUBERCULOSIS

T- ball
is
Ghon!

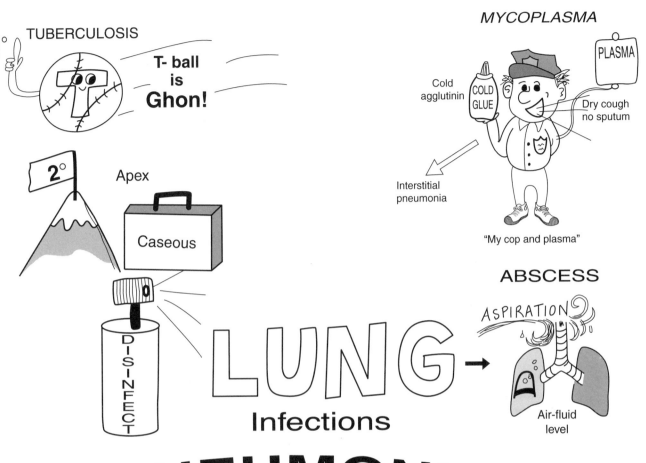

MYCOPLASMA

PLASMA

Cold
agglutinin

COLD
GLUE

Dry cough
no sputum

Interstitial
pneumonia

"My cop and plasma"

2°

Apex

Caseous

ABSCESS

ASPIRATION

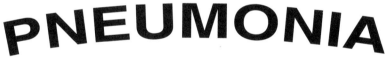

LUNG →
Infections

Air-fluid
level

D
I
S
I
N
F
E
C
T

PNEUMONIA

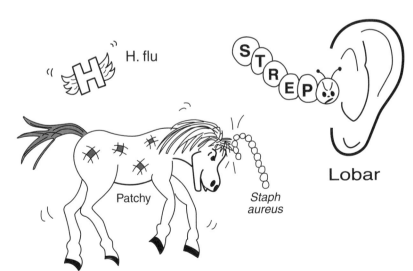

H. flu

STREP

Lobar

Staph
aureus

Patchy

Bronchopneumonia

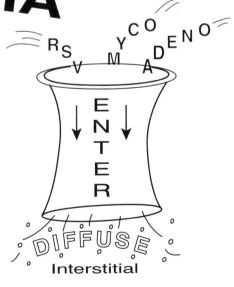

R S V M Y C O A D E N O

E
N
T
E
R

DIFFUSE
Interstitial

4.
BLOOD

NOTES

MICROCYTIC ANEMIAS

Iron Deficiency Anemia

⇒ "We need iron!"
- most common anemia
- insufficient iron supply to incorporate into red blood cell (RBC) hemoglobin (Hgb)
- causes include heavy menses, blood loss (gastrointestinal bleed), and dietary insufficiency, especially in children
- laboratory tests: ↓ serum iron, ↑ total iron-binding capacity (TIBC), ↓ ferritin, ↓ iron in bone marrow
- blood smear shows microcytosis and hypochromia (resulting in large pale centers) of RBCs

Sideroblastic Anemia

⇒ "This will cause a con**SIDER**able **BLAST**!"
- acquired or X-linked inheritance
  ⇒ X shape of dynamite
- defective heme synthase interferes with production of heme protein
- iron collects in body tissues; therefore, elevated serum iron
- iron stain (Prussian blue) of bone marrow reveals ringed sideroblasts (normoblast that contains ferritin, which reacts to Prussian blue stain, indicating that the iron is ionized and not attached to a heme group)
- laboratory tests: ↑ serum iron, ↑ TIBC, ↑ serum ferritin, ↑ iron in bone marrow

Thalassemia

⇒ "THA LASS SEEMS…"
- defective production of α- or β-Hgb chain; therefore, HgbA is unable to develop. (⇒ HgbA falling out of backpack); other hemoglobins such as $HgbA_2$ and HgbF form to compensate

Chronic Disease

⇒ watch spinning continuously
- in the early phase, anemia associated with chronic disease is normocytic normochromic; it becomes microcytic later when bone marrow cannot compensate for the iron deficiency (reticuloendothelial iron stores cannot be released)
- laboratory tests: ↓ serum iron, ↓ TIBC, ↑ ferritin, ↑ iron in bone marrow

Lead Poisoning

⇒ "This pencil **lead** to **poisoning**."
- lead inhibition of heme and globin production
- symptoms include seizures, encephalopathy, wrist and foot drop, renal tubular acidosis, ataxic gait, and Bruton's lines (bluish gumlines)
- RBC basophilic stippling
- treatment includes dimercaprol

Hereditary Spherocytosis

⇒ "I think he **INHERITED** your **SPHERICAL** shape."
- autosomal dominant inheritance
- hemolysis in spleen due to RBC membrane cytoskeleton irregularity
- positive osmotic fragility test

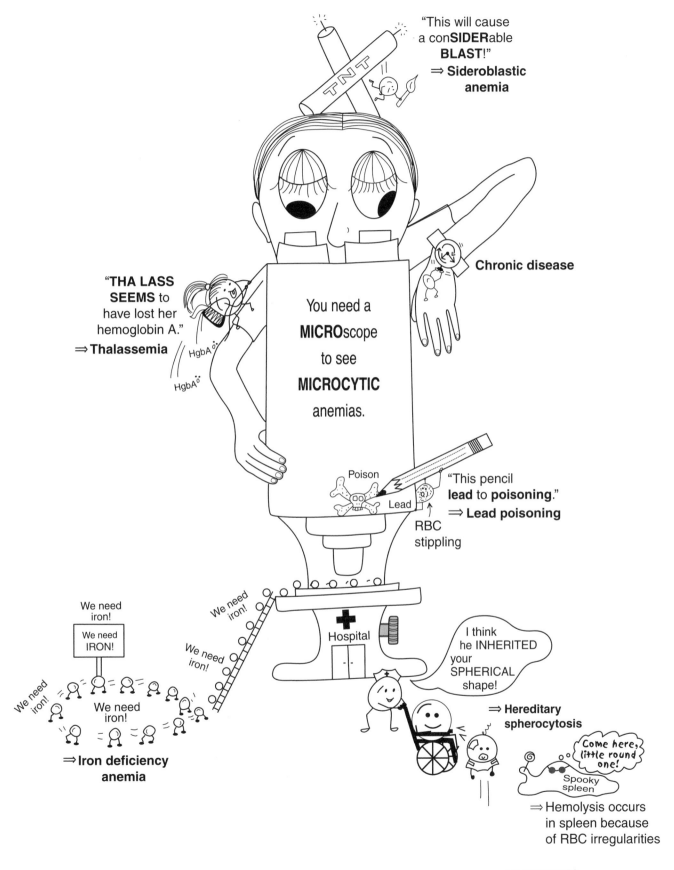

NOTES

MACROCYTIC ANEMIAS

Antimetabolite Drugs

- such as 5-fluorouracil⇒"5 flowers"

Alcoholism

- hemoglobin synthesis is disrupted in the bone marrow

Spur Cell Anemia

⇒ spurs on boots
- causes include alcoholic and viral hepatitis and liver cirrhosis
- RBC surface area is increased due to incorporation of cholesterol into RBC membranes

B_{12} Deficiency

⇒ Big Mac sitting on B_{12}
- nuclear maturation is delayed
- causes include pernicious anemia, acquired deficiency of intrinsic factor (gastrectomy), decreased absorption as occurs with ileal resection, and tapeworm (*Diphyllobothrium latum*), which uses B_{12}, thereby causing a deficiency
- symptoms include defective myelin synthesis, which causes neuropathies
- detected with Schilling test, which can determine origin of B_{12} deficiency
- treatment is parenteral B_{12}

Folic Acid Deficiency

⇒ Big Mac sitting on foal licking acid
- nuclear maturation is delayed
- primary cause is dietary deficiency, but it can also be caused by increased need for folate that occurs in pregnancy and alcoholism
- treatment always includes folate + B_{12} (B_{12} deficiency neurologic symptoms can only be corrected with B_{12})

Glucose-6-Phosphate Dehydrogenase (G6PD) Deficiency

⇒ Big Mac smashing G6PD with boot
- X-linked inheritance
- RBC lysis from oxidizing agents such as fava beans and oxidizing drugs
- Heinz bodies
- peripheral smear reveals reticulocytes (which are larger than normal mature RBCs) and hemolysis

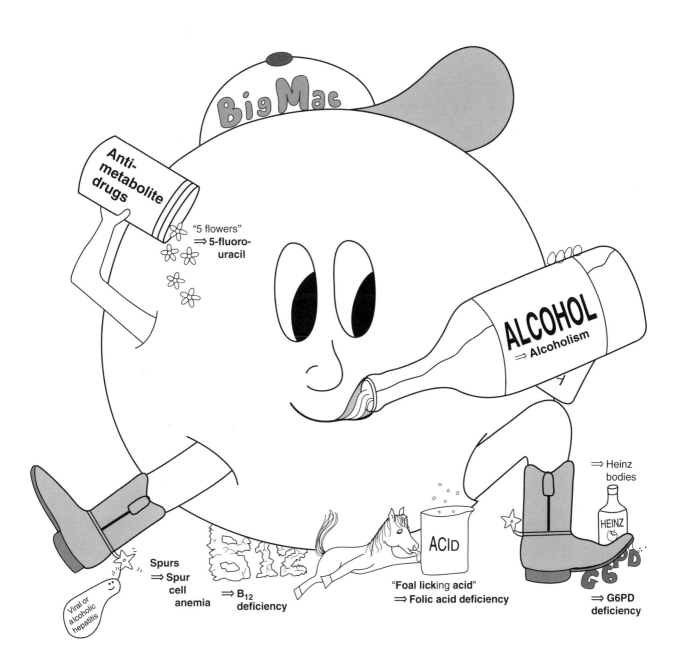

Big Mac

Anti-metabolite drugs

"5 flowers"
⇒ 5-fluoro-uracil

ALCOHOL
⇒ Alcoholism

⇒ Heinz bodies

HEINZ

G6PD

Viral or alcoholic hepatitis

Spurs
⇒ Spur cell anemia

⇒ B₁₂ deficiency

ACID

"Foal licking acid"
⇒ Folic acid deficiency

⇒ G6PD deficiency

NOTES

Aplastic Anemia

- drug-induced includes arsenic and chemotherapy
- infiltrative includes cancers of the bone such as leukemia
- pancytopenia

Hemolytic Anemia

- paroxysmal nocturnal hemoglobinuria, pyruvate kinase deficiency, sickle cell anemia, and so forth

Myelophthisic Anemia

- causes include infiltrative tumors that replace bone marrow with neoplasm
- extramedullary erythropoiesis
- blood smear reveals teardrop cells

RBC Aplasia

- RBCs are only cell line affected by autoimmune process or B19 (parvovirus) infection

Acute Hemorrhagic Anemia

- acute, rapid, and severe bleeding can lead to hypovolemic shock

Hypoproliferative Anemia

- ↓ erythropoietin from chronic renal disease

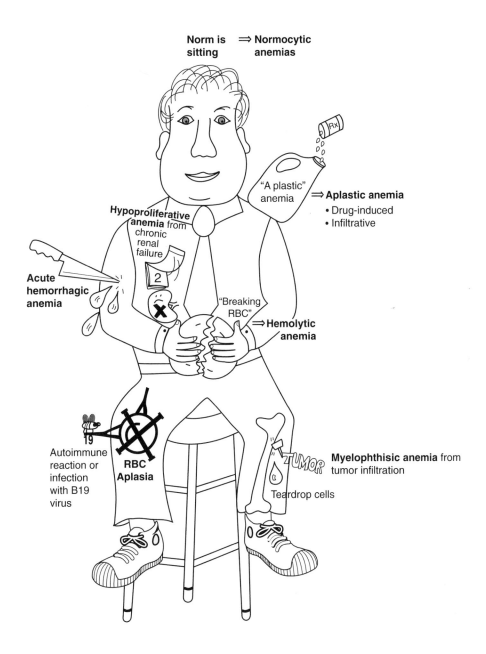

Norm is sitting ⇒ Normocytic anemias

"A plastic" anemia ⇒ **Aplastic anemia**
- Drug-induced
- Infiltrative

Hypoproliferative anemia from chronic renal failure

Acute hemorrhagic anemia

"Breaking RBC" ⇒ **Hemolytic anemia**

Autoimmune reaction or infection with B19 virus

RBC Aplasia

Myelophthisic anemia from tumor infiltration

Teardrop cells

SICKLE CELL ANEMIA

- single valine amino acid substitution for glutamic acid on beta chain
- RBCs crescent or sickle shaped
- homozygote complications include vaso-occlusive crisis, autosplenectomy, infection with encapsulated organisms, aplastic anemia from B19 parvovirus infection (further suppression of already low RBC production), and *Salmonella* osteomyelitis
- treatment includes hydroxyurea and bone marrow transplant

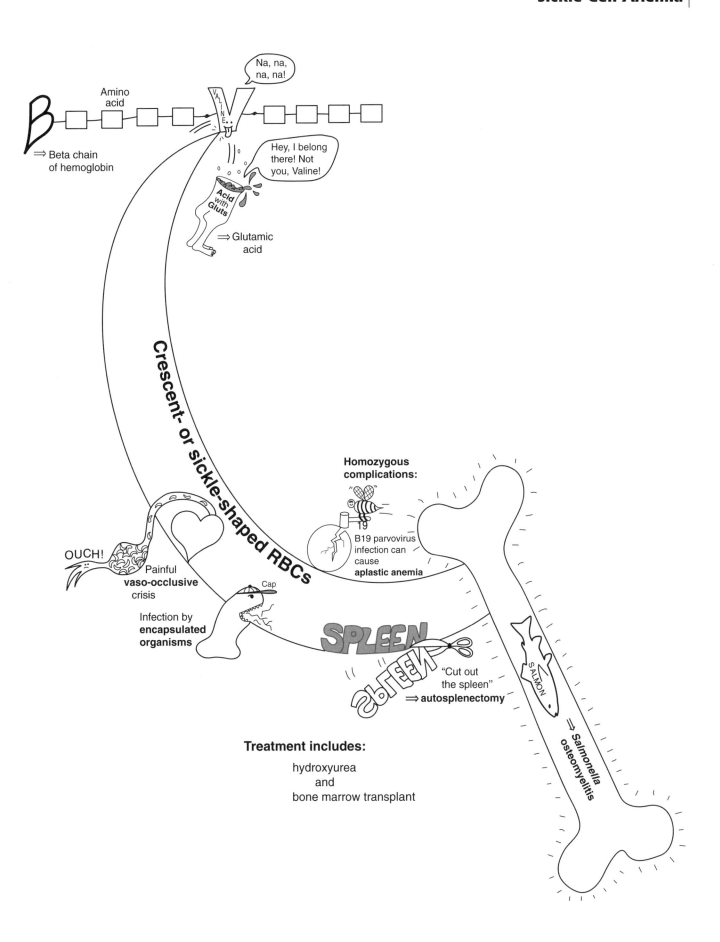

NOTES

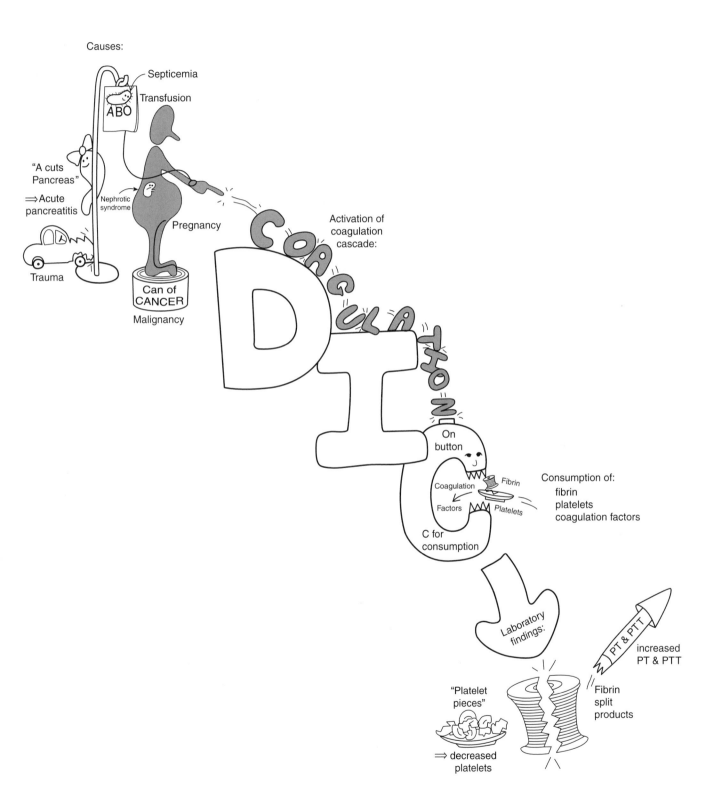

Causes:

Septicemia

Transfusion

ABO

"A cuts Pancreas"

⟹Acute pancreatitis

Nephrotic syndrome

Trauma

Pregnancy

Can of CANCER

Malignancy

Activation of coagulation cascade:

On button

Coagulation Fibrin

Factors Platelets

C for consumption

Consumption of:
fibrin
platelets
coagulation factors

Laboratory findings:

"Platelet pieces"

⟹ decreased platelets

Fibrin split products

PT & PTT

increased PT & PTT

NOTES

THROMBOTIC THROMBOCYTIC PURPURA (TTP)

Pathogenesis

- antibodies to endothelial cells cause platelet-fibrin thrombi in capillaries
- peripheral smear shows schistocytes (fragmented RBCs)

Pentad of TTP

- neurologic changes
- fever
- thrombocytopenia
- renal failure leads to ↑ creatinine, hematuria, and proteinuria
- intravascular hemolytic anemia

Treatment

- IV immunoglobulin (Ig) or plasma exchange

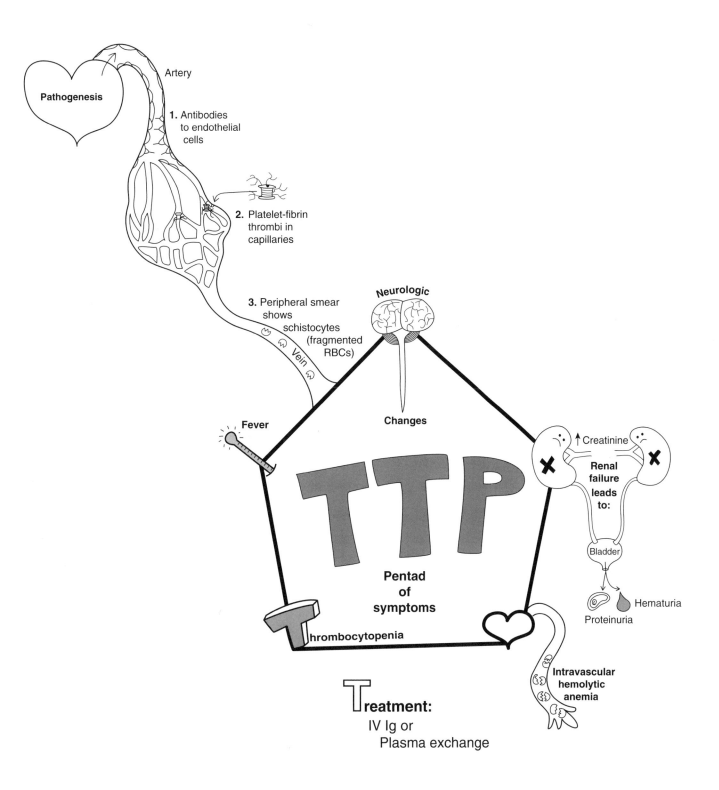

Pathogenesis

Artery

1. Antibodies to endothelial cells

2. Platelet-fibrin thrombi in capillaries

3. Peripheral smear shows schistocytes (fragmented RBCs)

Vein

Neurologic

Changes

Fever

TTP

Pentad of symptoms

↑Creatinine

Renal failure leads to:

Bladder

Hematuria

Proteinuria

Thrombocytopenia

Intravascular hemolytic anemia

Treatment:
IV Ig or
Plasma exchange

NOTES

LEUKEMIA

■ ACUTE LEUKEMIAS

- pancytopenia
- bone marrow failure with greater than 30% blasts in bone marrow
- occur in children or elderly
- smudge cells (occur with lymphocytic leukemias)—partially disintegrated cells

Acute Lymphocytic Leukemia

- children more commonly afflicted
- TdT marker
- lymphoblasts→immature B cells
- therapy most effective
- associated with Down syndrome

Acute Myeloid Leukemia

- M3 (promyelocytic leukemia) associated with DIC and Auer bodies
- no TdT marker
- myeloblasts
- more common in adults

■ CHRONIC LEUKEMIAS

- mature cells involved more often
- more common in the elderly
- longer course when compared to acute leukemias

Chronic Lymphocytic Leukemia

- mature B cells involved that are non–antibody generating (hypoglobulinemia)
- same B-cell markers as small lymphocytic lymphoma (CD19/CD5 markers)
- autoimmune hemolytic anemia
- elderly
- lymphadenopathy and hepatosplenomegaly

Chronic Myeloid Leukemia

- associated with Philadelphia chromosome
- t(9;22); *bcr-abl*
- blast crisis→myeloid stem cell proliferation
- leukocytosis and thrombocytosis
- splenomegaly

Lymphocytic
Acute lymphocytic leukemia (ALL)

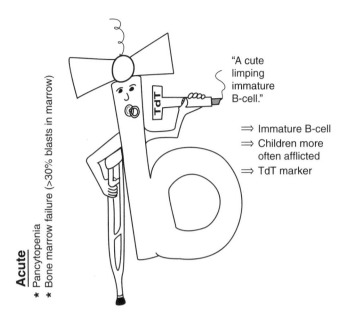

"A cute limping immature B-cell."

$\Rightarrow$ Immature B-cell
$\Rightarrow$ Children more often afflicted
$\Rightarrow$ TdT marker

Acute
* Pancytopenia
* Bone marrow failure (>30% blasts in marrow)

Myelocytic
Acute myeloid leukemia (AML)

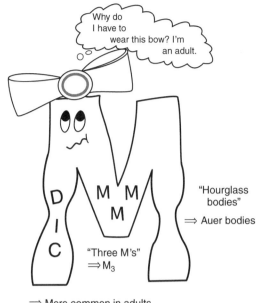

Why do I have to wear this bow? I'm an adult.

"Hourglass bodies"
$\Rightarrow$ Auer bodies

"Three M's"
$\Rightarrow M_3$

$\Rightarrow$ More common in adults
$\Rightarrow M_3$ (Promyelocytic leukemia) is associated with Auer bodies and DIC
$\Rightarrow$ No TdT marker as in ALL

Chronic lymphocytic leukemia (CLL)

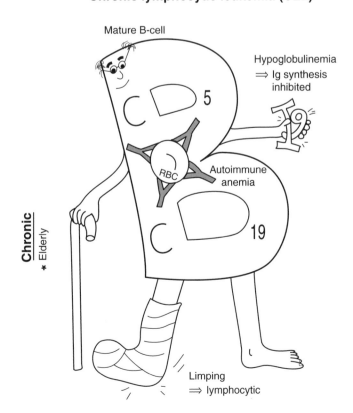

Mature B-cell

Hypoglobulinemia
$\Rightarrow$ Ig synthesis inhibited

5

RBC

Autoimmune anemia

19

Limping
$\Rightarrow$ lymphocytic

Chronic
* Elderly

Chronic myeloid leukemia (CML)

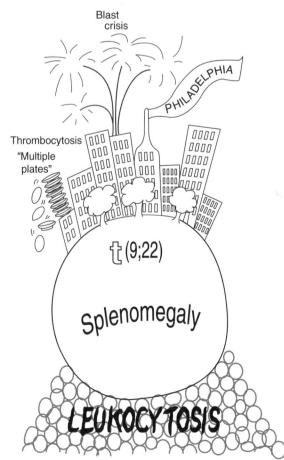

Blast crisis

PHILADELPHIA

Thrombocytosis
"Multiple plates"

t (9;22)

Splenomegaly

LEUKOCYTOSIS

NOTES

MULTIPLE MYELOMA

- number one adult primary bone tumor
- monoclonal plasma cell cancer
- large amounts of IgG and IgA produced
- hypercalcemia
- renal insufficiency
- increased risk of infection
- anemia
- punched-out lytic bone lesions on x-ray
- M-spike on serum protein electrophoresis
- Bence Jones proteins in urine (Ig light chains)
- rouleau (stacked) formation of RBCs

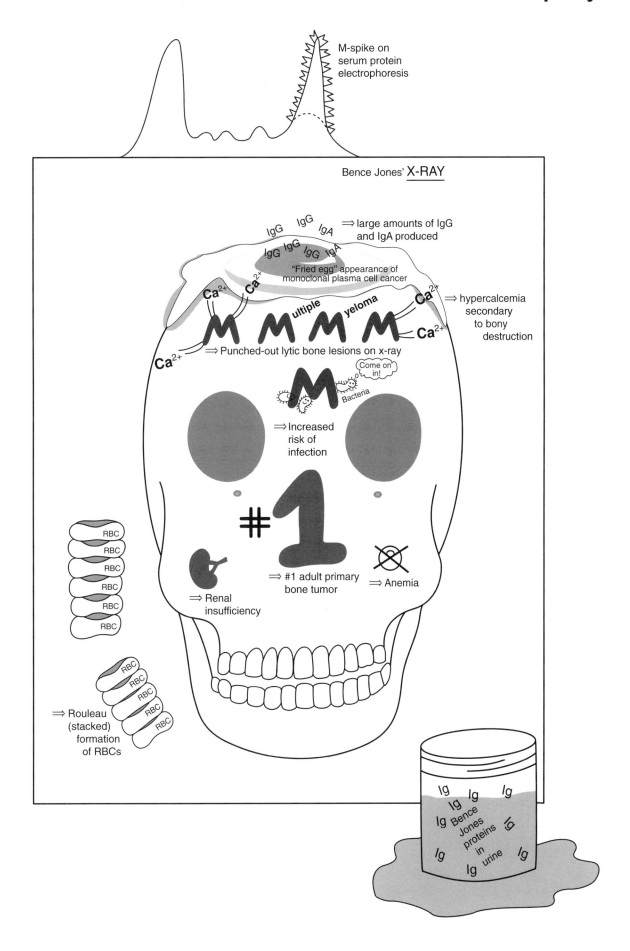

M-spike on serum protein electrophoresis

Bence Jones' X-RAY

⇒ large amounts of IgG and IgA produced

"Fried egg" appearance of monoclonal plasma cell cancer

⇒ hypercalcemia secondary to bony destruction

⇒ Punched-out lytic bone lesions on x-ray

Come on in!

Bacteria

⇒ Increased risk of infection

#1

⇒ #1 adult primary bone tumor

⇒ Anemia

⇒ Renal insufficiency

⇒ Rouleau (stacked) formation of RBCs

Ig Bence Jones proteins in urine

5.
GASTROINTESTINAL TRACT

NOTES

NOTES

Plummer-Vinson syndrome

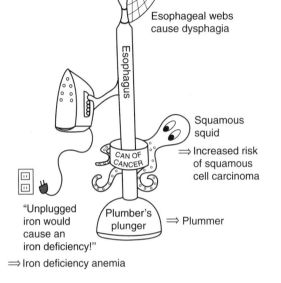

Deer = venison = Vinson

Glossitis

Esophageal webs
cause dysphagia

Esophagus

CAN OF CANCER

Squamous
squid

⇒ Increased risk
of squamous
cell carcinoma

"Unplugged
iron would
cause an
iron deficiency!"

⇒ Iron deficiency anemia

Plumber's
plunger ⇒ Plummer

Achalasia

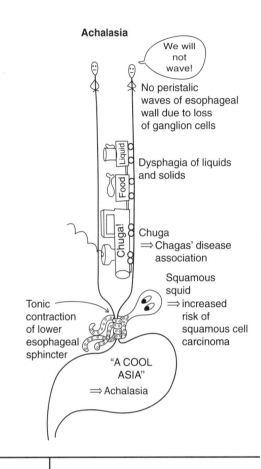

We will
not
wave!

No peristalic
waves of esophageal
wall due to loss
of ganglion cells

Liquid

Dysphagia of liquids
and solids

Food

Chuga!

Chuga
⇒ Chagas' disease
association

Tonic
contraction
of lower
esophageal
sphincter

Squamous
squid
⇒ increased
risk of
squamous cell
carcinoma

"A COOL
ASIA"

⇒ Achalasia

Zenker's diverticulum

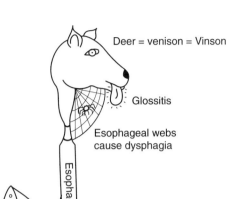

I
think I
got a big
one!

Zenker
sinker

Occurs in
⇒ upper
esophagus

Mallory-Weiss syndrome
⇒ Mallory wise

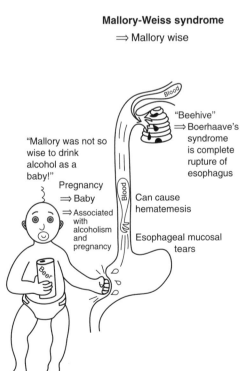

Blood

"Beehive"
⇒ Boerhaave's
syndrome
is complete
rupture of
esophagus

"Mallory was not so
wise to drink
alcohol as a
baby!"

Blood

Can cause
hematemesis

Pregnancy
⇒ Baby

⇒ Associated
with
alcoholism
and
pregnancy

Esophageal mucosal
tears

Beer

Esophageal varices

Blood

Painless
hematemesis

Blood

Dilation of
submucosal
vein in
esophagus

Portal hypertension
is primary cause

Liver

NOTES

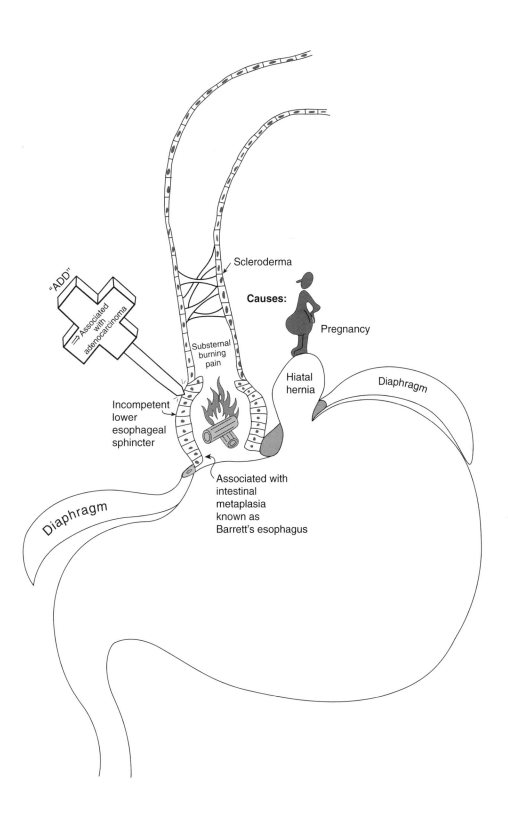

"ADD"

⇒ Associated with adenocarcinoma

Scleroderma

Causes:

Pregnancy

Substernal burning pain

Incompetent lower esophageal sphincter

Hiatal hernia

Diaphragm

Associated with intestinal metaplasia known as Barrett's esophagus

Diaphragm

NOTES

CHRONIC GASTRITIS

- ⇒ gas pump holding clock (chronic)
- increased risk of gastric carcinoma
- ⇒ can of CANCER

Type A = Fundal

- ⇒ fun A
- autoimmune process
- caused by autoantibodies to parietal cells that produce intrinsic factor and HCl
    - ⇒ automobile hitting pair of eyes
- leads to pernicious anemia (vitamin B_{12} deficiency) and achlorhydria (absence of free HCl)
    - ⇒ bees with perms and HCl running away
- increased risk of gastric adenocarcinoma

Type B = Antral

- ⇒ B with ants
- caused by *Helicobacter pylori* infection
    - ⇒ helicopter with pie
- most common gastritis
- complications include chronic ulcers, gastric adenocarcinoma, and gastric lymphoma

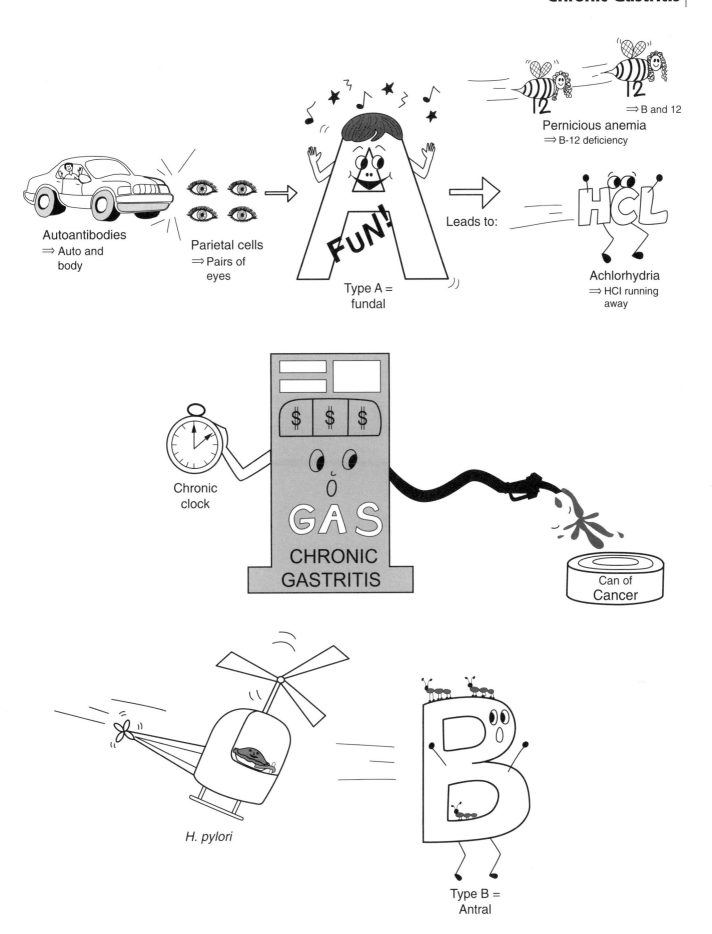

Autoantibodies
⇒ Auto and body

Parietal cells
⇒ Pairs of eyes

Type A = fundal

Leads to:

Pernicious anemia
⇒ B-12 deficiency

⇒ B and 12

Achlorhydria
⇒ HCl running away

Chronic clock

GAS
CHRONIC GASTRITIS

Can of Cancer

H. pylori

Type B = Antral

PEPTIC ULCER DISEASE (PUD)

⇒ peppy tick
- consequences of PUD include hemorrhage, perforation, and obstruction

Gastric Ulcer (25% of Ulcers)

⇒ gas pump
- involves decreased mucosal protection to acid or *H. pylori*
  ⇒ gas pump squishing mucosa
- caused by *H. pylori* (70%), nonsteroidal anti-inflammatory drugs (NSAIDs), caffeine, cigarette smoking
  ⇒ bottle of aspirin smoking a cigarette
- pain increases with eating
  ⇒ gas pump holding tummy
- commonly affects antral and prepyloric areas
- normal to low acid production
  ⇒ small jar of acid

Duodenal Ulcer (75% of Ulcers)

⇒ singing duo
- due to increased gastric acid secretion
  ⇒ big jar of acid
- caused by *H. pylori* (most common), NSAIDs, blood type O, caffeine, cigarette smoking, Zollinger-Ellison syndrome
  ⇒ aspirin and cigarette
- pain decreases with eating
  ⇒ duo eating
- hypertrophy of Brunner's glands, which secrete alkaline mucus and are located in the submucosa

H. pylori infection can be treated with metronidazole, bismuth salicylate, amoxicillin, and a proton pump inhibitor
⇒ helicopter with pie, Metro bus, "Bismuth or bust," and ox driving bus

Cushing's Ulcer

- associated with central nervous system (CNS) trauma
  ⇒ brain on a cushion

Curling's Ulcer

- associated with burn injury
  ⇒ hot curling iron

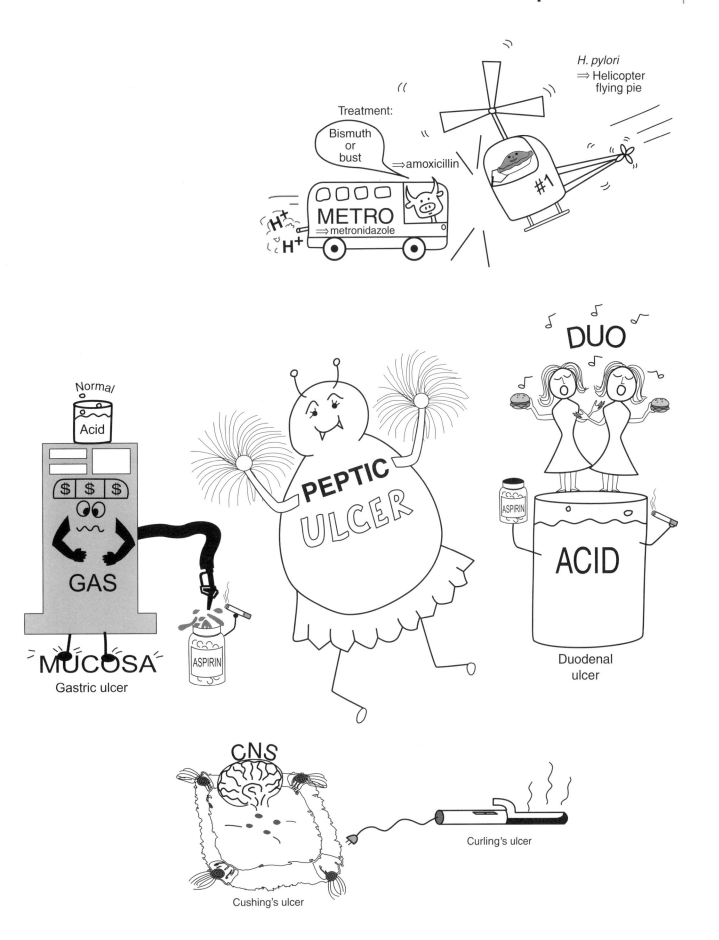

Gastric ulcer

Duodenal ulcer

Cushing's ulcer

Curling's ulcer

STOMACH TUMORS

⇒ tomb with stomach on it

Gastric Adenocarcinoma

⇒ stomach with "ADD IN NO" sign on can of CANCER

• antral and prepyloric areas most affected

• patients present with weight loss and satiety

• early metastasis to lymph nodes and liver

• related to chronic gastritis type B and exposure to nitrites in food preservatives (smoked fish)

⇒ gas pump and fish bone

• metastasis to the supraclavicular nodes is known as a *Virchow's node*

• Krukenberg's tumor metastasizes to ovaries

⇒ crooked line to eggs

• signet ring cells present and stains positive for mucin

⇒ ring and facial tissue box

Gastric Lymphoma

⇒ phone on a limb

• caused by *H. pylori*

⇒ pie in a helicopter

• low grade has lymphoid tissue in mucosa

• high grade associated with B-cell lymphoma

• incidence increased in patients with acquired immunodeficiency syndrome (AIDS)

• stains negative for mucin

⇒ crossed-out facial tissue box

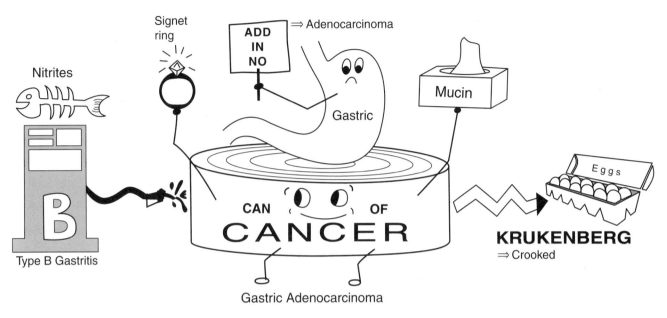

Nitrites

Signet ring

⇒ Adenocarcinoma

ADD IN NO

Gastric

Mucin

Eggs

B

Type B Gastritis

CAN OF
CANCER

Gastric Adenocarcinoma

KRUKENBERG
⇒ Crooked

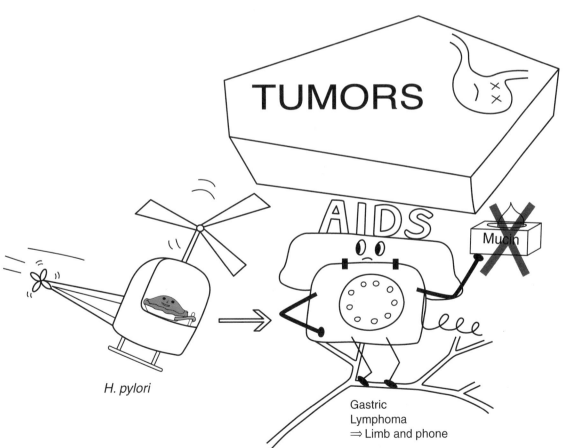

TUMORS

AIDS

Mucin

H. pylori

Gastric
Lymphoma
⇒ Limb and phone

NOTES

INFLAMMATORY BOWEL DISEASE

⇒ bowl in flames
- characteristics include fever, chronic bloody diarrhea, uveitis iritis, and aphthous ulcers
  - ⇒ thermometer, bloody toilet paper, and big irritated eyes
- more common among Jews, affects whites more than blacks

Ulcerative Colitis

⇒ coal with ulcer
- occurs more often in women than in men
- involves the colon and rectum
- continuous lesion
  - ⇒ continuous arrow around coal
- pseudopolyps form after ulcers re-epithelialize
  - ⇒ lips on coal
- crypt abscesses seen microscopically
  - ⇒ coal standing on crypt
- complications include toxic megacolon and colorectal adenocarcinoma (risk = 25×)
  - ⇒ skull and crossbones and can of CANCER

Crohn's Disease

⇒ crown
- occurs with equal frequency in men and women
- involves gastrointestinal tract, most commonly the terminal ileum; rectal sparing
- skip lesions are patchy lesions of ulcerated mucosa
  - ⇒ crown skipping rope
- intestinal wall thickening gives a lead pipe appearance known as a *string sign* on x-ray
  - ⇒ thick rope
- transmural inflammation, cobblestone mucosa, and creeping fat seen on examination
  - ⇒ cobblestone road and crawling butter
- noncaseating granulomas seen microscopically
  - ⇒ case with granny crossed out
- complications include fistulas, strictures, perianal disease, and weight loss
  - ⇒ crown has big fists

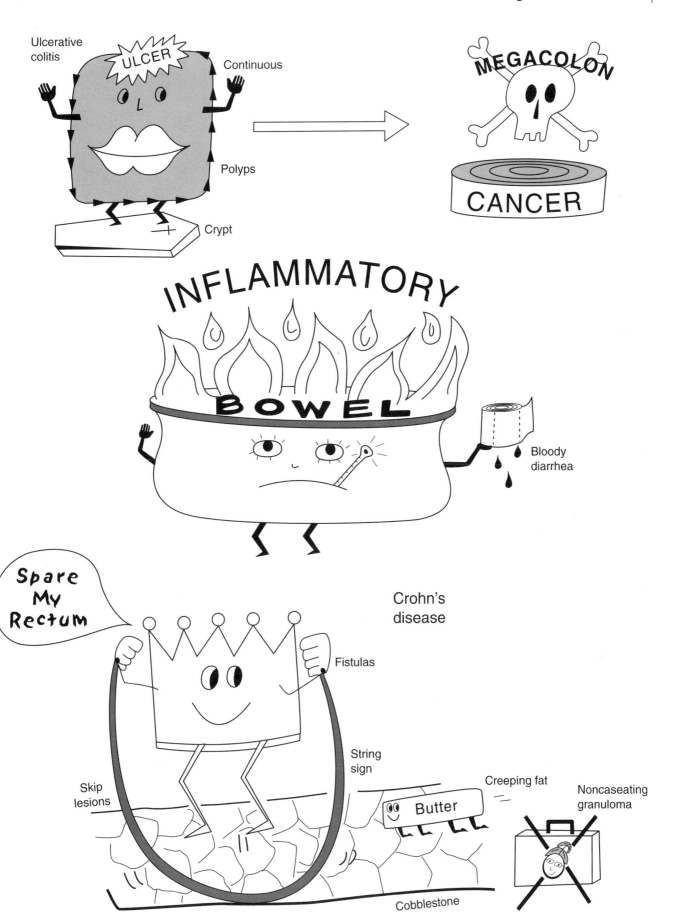

NOTES

DIVERTICULAR DISEASE

⇒ diver

Diverticulum

- blind pouch where only the mucosa herniates
- usually located in the sigmoid colon
  ⇒ bottle of sigmoid cologne
- caused by low-fiber diet and high intraluminal pressures during defecation
- saw-toothed appearance on barium enema (BE)
  ⇒ saw in diver's hand

Diverticulosis

- many diverticula
- patients present in their 60s
  ⇒ 60 on diver's back
- complications include obstruction or perforation
  ⇒ construction obstruction barrier

Diverticulitis

- inflammation of diverticulum
- causes left lower quadrant (LLQ) pain, fever, and bloody stools
  ⇒ thermometer and toilet paper with blood droplets
- complications include perforation, abscesses, and peritonitis
- treatment includes high-fiber diet

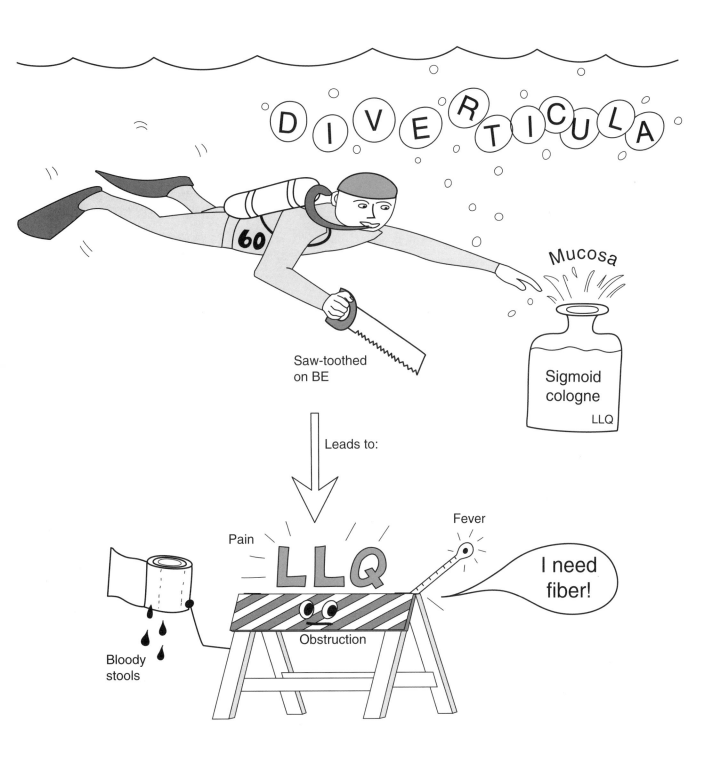

INTESTINAL POLYPS

⇒ lips on a pole

Nonneoplastic Polyps

- hyperplastic polyps are the most common type of benign polyp and asymptomatic with no increased risk of carcinoma
- pseudopolyps are inflammatory and seen in ulcerative colitis

Adenomatous Polyps

- tubular adenomas are the most common type: asymptomatic, small, premalignant, and on a thin stalk
⇒ tuba on a stem making number one sign
    - composed of neoplastic glands with or without mucin
    - may have occult bleeding
- villous adenomas are uncommon (<10%), asymptomatic, larger, most malignant, and without a stalk
⇒ big gun
    - composed of neoplastic epithelium
    - may have occult bleeding

Polyposis Syndromes

- familial adenomatous polyposis (FAP) is the most common type, autosomal dominant, and appears in young adulthood
    ⇒ FAP making number one sign
    - risk for malignancy is 100%
    ⇒ can of CANCER
    - main symptom is rectal bleeding
- Gardner's syndrome is autosomal dominant and causes adenomatous polyps
    ⇒ man in garden
    - associated with fibromas and osteomas in other tissues
    ⇒ bones in garden
    - risk for malignancy is 100%
- Turcot's syndrome is autosomal recessive and causes adenomatous polyps in the colon
    ⇒ turkey on a cot
    - associated with astrocytoma
    ⇒ asteroid
    - risk for malignancy is 100%
- Peutz-Jeghers syndrome is autosomal dominant and causes benign hamartomatous polyps in the small intestine
⇒ jug holding nose saying "Pee-U" and hammer on toe
    - melanin pigmentation of oral mucosa, lips, hands, and genitalia
    ⇒ darkened hands and lips
    - increased incidence of breast, ovarian, and stomach cancer

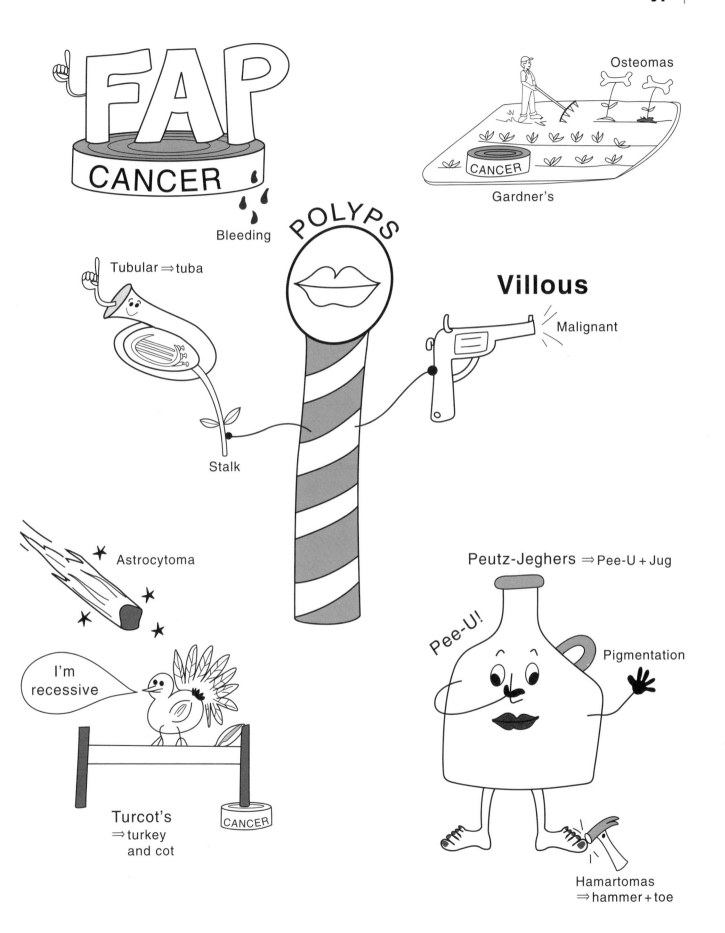

Osteomas

Gardner's

FAP
CANCER
Bleeding

POLYPS

Tubular ⇒ tuba

Villous

Malignant

Stalk

Astrocytoma

Peutz-Jeghers ⇒ Pee-U + Jug

Pee-U!

Pigmentation

I'm recessive

Turcot's
⇒ turkey and cot

CANCER

Hamartomas
⇒ hammer + toe

NOTES

INTESTINAL TUMORS

⇒ tomb with intestine on it

Colorectal Adenocarcinoma

⇒ cologne on can of CANCER
- most common malignancy of gastrointestinal tract
- associated with adenomatous polyps, ulcerative colitis, low-fiber diet, high-fat diet, and family history
  ⇒ lips and butter
- elevated carcinoembryonic antigen (CEA)
- right-sided tumor (cecal) presents with weight loss and iron-deficiency anemia
  ⇒ iron
- left-sided tumor (colorectal) presents with occult bleeding and changes in bowel habits
  ⇒ toilet paper with blood droplets

Small Intestine Adenocarcinoma

⇒ "add in no": sign
- associated with Crohn's disease
  ⇒ crowns
- occurs most commonly in duodenum
  ⇒ singing duo

Carcinoid Tumor

⇒ car
- occurs most commonly in appendix (benign)
- may be benign or malignant
- symptoms of carcinoid syndrome include watery diarrhea, flushing, and bronchospasm
  ⇒ flushing face, cough, and water out of tailpipe

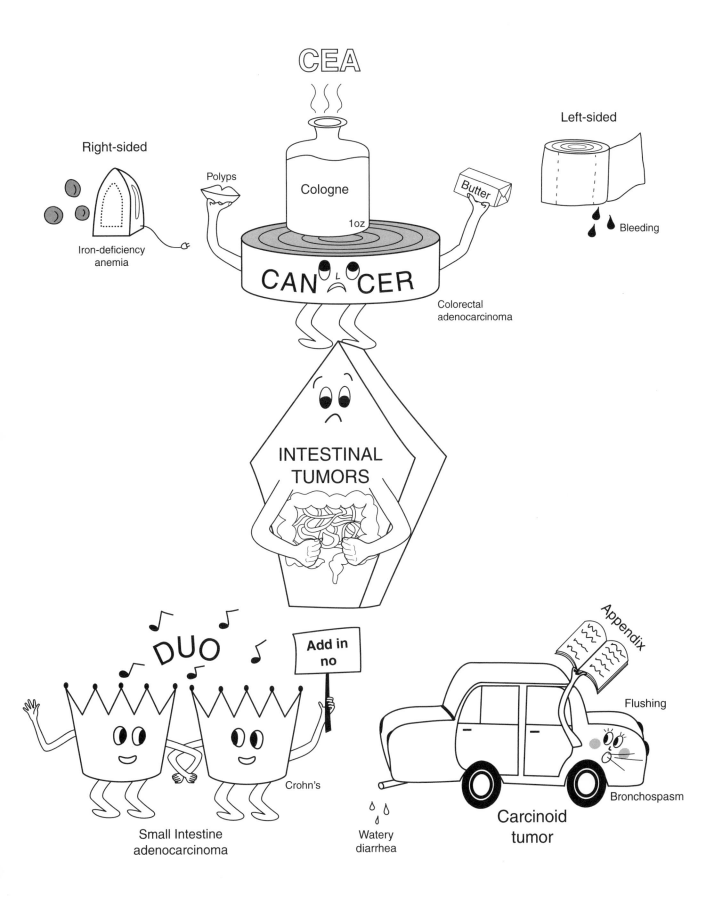

CEA

Right-sided

Iron-deficiency anemia

Polyps

Cologne

1oz

CAN CER

Colorectal adenocarcinoma

Left-sided

Butter

Bleeding

INTESTINAL TUMORS

DUO

Add in no

Crohn's

Small Intestine adenocarcinoma

Watery diarrhea

Appendix

Flushing

Bronchospasm

Carcinoid tumor

NOTES

BOWEL OBSTRUCTION

⇒ bowl on construction obstruction barrier

Hernias

⇒ her knee
- can cause bowel ischemia or strangulation

Direct inguinal hernias protrude through the abdominal wall and through the external ring of the inguinal canal
⇒ solid arrow and ring in man's hand
- usually occur in older men
  ⇒ old man with cane
- enter medial to inferior epigastric artery

Indirect inguinal hernias enter the internal ring and external ring of the inguinal canal and can enter the scrotum
⇒ segmented arrow and two rings being kicked and baby holding scrotum
- enter internal ring lateral to inferior epigastric artery
- caused by patent processus vaginalis
- most common hernia in males and infants
  ⇒ baby makes number one sign

Femoral hernias protrude into the femoral canal below the inguinal ligament

Other types of hernias include incisional, hiatal, and umbilical

Volvulus

⇒ twisting tornado
- twisting of bowel loop
- usually occurs in the sigmoid colon
- causes abdominal pain, bowel ischemia, and strangulation

Intussusception

- a segment of bowel telescopes into another segment
  ⇒ telescope
- most often at the ileocecal junction
  ⇒ ileocecal junction sign
- may cause abdominal pain, vomiting, and rectal bleeding

Hirschsprung's Disease

⇒ girl spring
- absence of parasympathetic ganglion cells leads to congenital megacolon
  ⇒ "Where's my ganglion?"
- colon is dilated proximal to the aganglionic segment
  ⇒ dilated spring

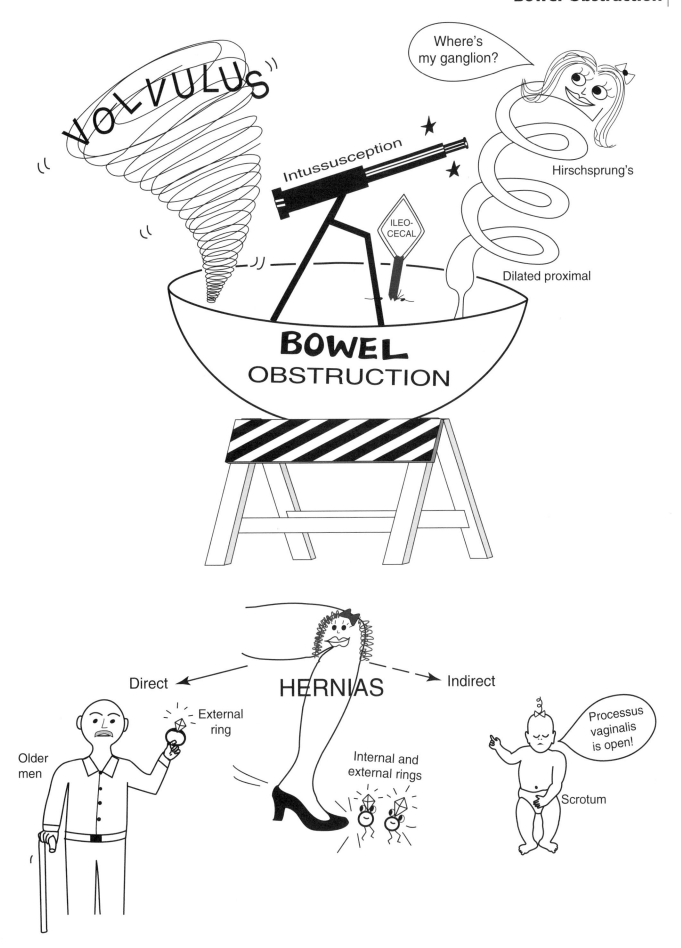

NOTES

MALABSORPTION SYNDROMES

⇒ sponge not absorbing

Celiac Disease

⇒ seal
- caused by eating gluten in wheat products
    ⇒ glue holding wheat
- leads to weight loss and diarrhea with pale stools
    ⇒ toilet paper
- blunting of small intestinal villi
    ⇒ seal squishing villi
- associated with intestinal T-cell lymphoma

Tropical Sprue

⇒ tropical tree
- caused by chronic bacterial infection of intestines
- vitamin B_{12} and folate malabsorption
    ⇒ bee and foal running away
- megaloblastic anemia develops
    ⇒ megaphone spitting out red blood cells
- blunting of small intestinal villi
    ⇒ tropical tree squishing villi

Whipple's Disease

⇒ whip
- para-aminosalicylic acid (PAS)-positive macrophage in intestinal mucosa
- leads to ascites, fever, and polyarthritis

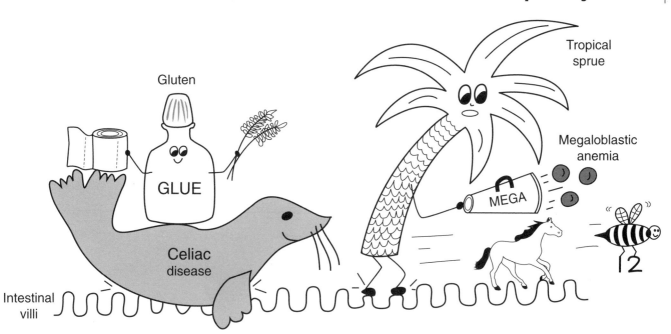

Gluten

Tropical sprue

Megaloblastic anemia

GLUE

MEGA

Celiac disease

Intestinal villi

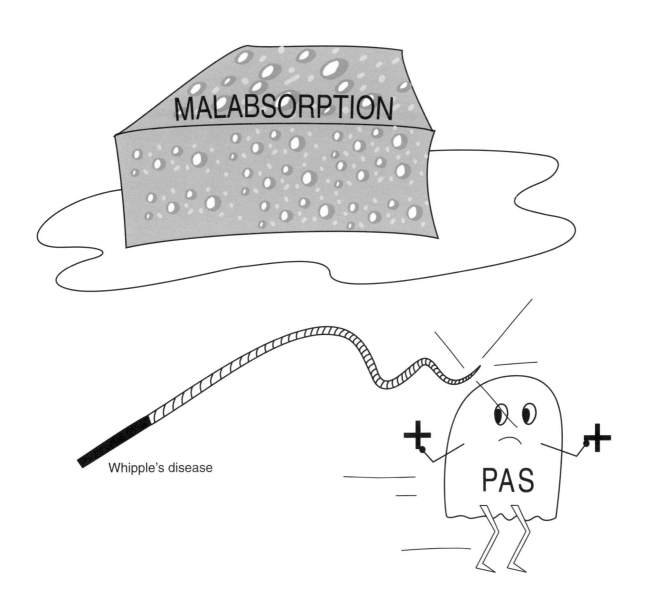

MALABSORPTION

Whipple's disease

PAS

6.
LIVER AND PANCREAS

CONGENITAL HYPERBILIRUBINEMIAS

⇒ hyper "belly rubbin'"

Crigler-Najjar Syndrome

⇒ Craig
- caused by a deficiency in glucuronyl transferase
- characterized by
  - increase in unconjugated bilirubin
  - ⇒ Craig and Gilbert unconnected to belly rubbin'
  - jaundice
  - ⇒ dice
  - kernicterus (bilirubin accumulation in the brain)
  - ⇒ kernels
- patients present early in life
- leads to an early death

Gilbert's Syndrome

⇒ Gilbert
- slight decrease in glucuronyl transferase and uptake
- increase in unconjugated bilirubin
- ⇒ Craig and Gilbert unconnected to belly rubbin'
- asymptomatic; no clinical consequences
- ⇒ "I'm okay"

Dubin-Johnson Syndrome

- caused by defective bilirubin excretion
- increase in conjugated bilirubin
- ⇒ Mr. Dubin and Mr. Johnson connected to belly rubbin'
- black discoloration of the liver
- ⇒ black shirts

Rotor Syndrome

- similar to Dubin-Johnson but does not cause black discoloration of the liver

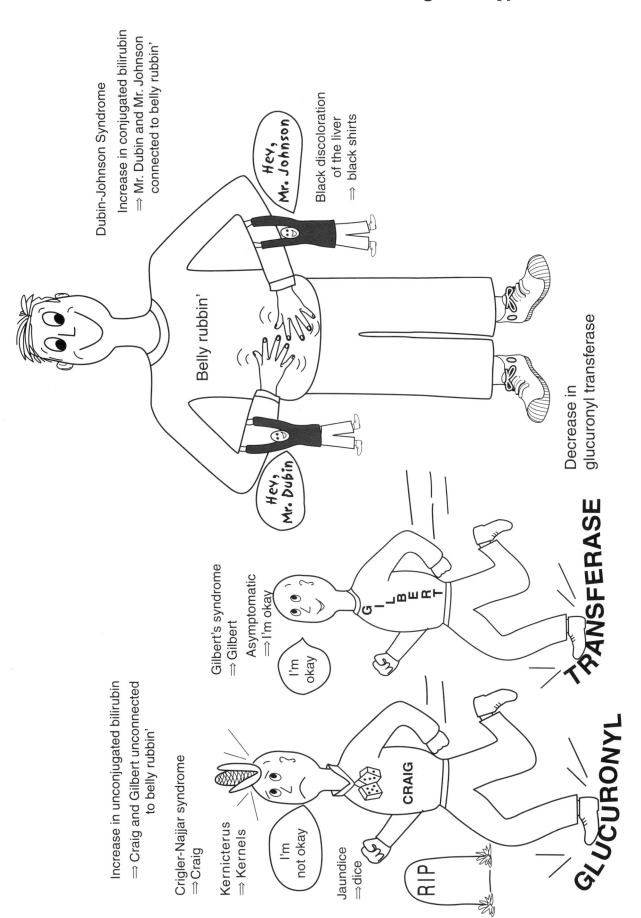

NOTES

CIRRHOSIS

⇒ Sir Hose

- chronic liver disease resulting in fibrosis and nodule formation
- increased risk of hepatocellular carcinoma
  - ⇒ can of CANCER
- causes include
  - excessive alcohol intake
  - ⇒ beer
  - hepatitis
  - ⇒ HEP
  - biliary obstruction
  - Wilson's disease
  - hemochromatosis
  - ⇒ crow
  - α_1-antitrypsin deficiency and other errors of metabolism
  - ⇒ no tripping
- clinical manifestations include
  - jaundice
  - ⇒ dice
  - peripheral edema
  - ⇒ swollen hand
  - spider nevi
  - gynecomastia
  - ⇒ male breasts
  - loss of body hair
  - asterixis (flapping hand tremor)
  - ⇒ asteroid hand tremor
  - coma
  - ⇒ sleeping face
  - coagulation factor deficiencies and anemia
  - portal hypertension (esophageal varices, splenomegaly, hemorrhoids, caput medusae)
  - ⇒ porthole HTN
- classification
  - micronodular (alcohol)
  - macronodular (hepatitis)

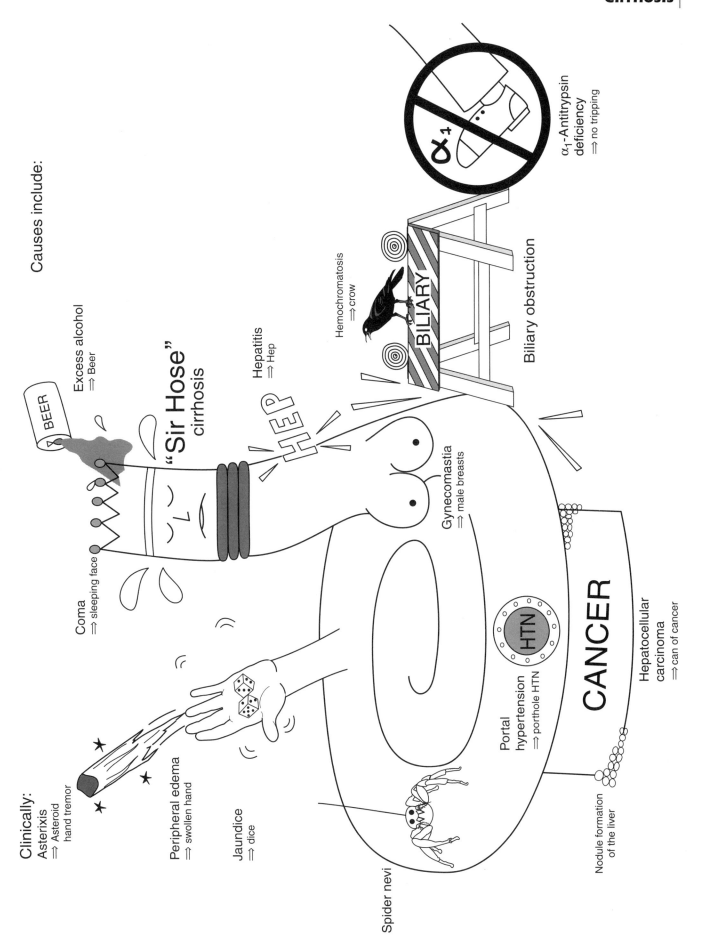

Causes include:

Excess alcohol
⇒ Beer

"Sir Hose"
cirrhosis

Hepatitis
⇒ Hep

Hemochromatosis
⇒ crow

BILIARY

Biliary obstruction

α₁-Antitrypsin
deficiency
⇒ no tripping

Clinically:
Asterixis
⇒ Asteroid
hand tremor

Coma
⇒ sleeping face

Peripheral edema
⇒ swollen hand

Gynecomastia
⇒ male breasts

Jaundice
⇒ dice

Spider nevi

Portal
hypertension
⇒ porthole HTN

HTN

CANCER

Hepatocellular
carcinoma
⇒ can of cancer

Nodule formation
of the liver

BEER

HEP

NOTES

WILSON'S DISEASE

⇒ Mr. Wilson the Cop
- disorder of copper metabolism due to autosomal recessive defect
- copper accumulates in the liver, brain, and cornea
  ⇒ cop and pennies
- also known as *hepatolenticular degeneration*
- characterized by
  - decreased ceruloplasmin (copper-binding protein)
  - cirrhosis
  ⇒ Sir Hose
  - Kayser-Fleischer rings (corneal deposits)
  ⇒ rings on hand
  ⇒ copper penny corneas
  - basal ganglia involvement
  ⇒ the basal gang
  - asterixis and choreiform movements
  ⇒ asterixis⇒asteroid and hand tremor; choreiform⇒dancing
  - treatment includes penicillamine
  ⇒ pencil

Basal ganglia
Degeneration
⇒ The basal gang

Treatment: Penicillamine

Kayser-Fleischer rings
⇒ rings on hand
⇒ copper penny
corneas

Copper
accumulation
⇒ cop and
pennies

Cirrhosis
⇒ Sir Hose

Asterixis
⇒ Asteroid
⇒ Hand tremor

Choreiform movement
⇒ Dancing

Decreased ceruloplasmin

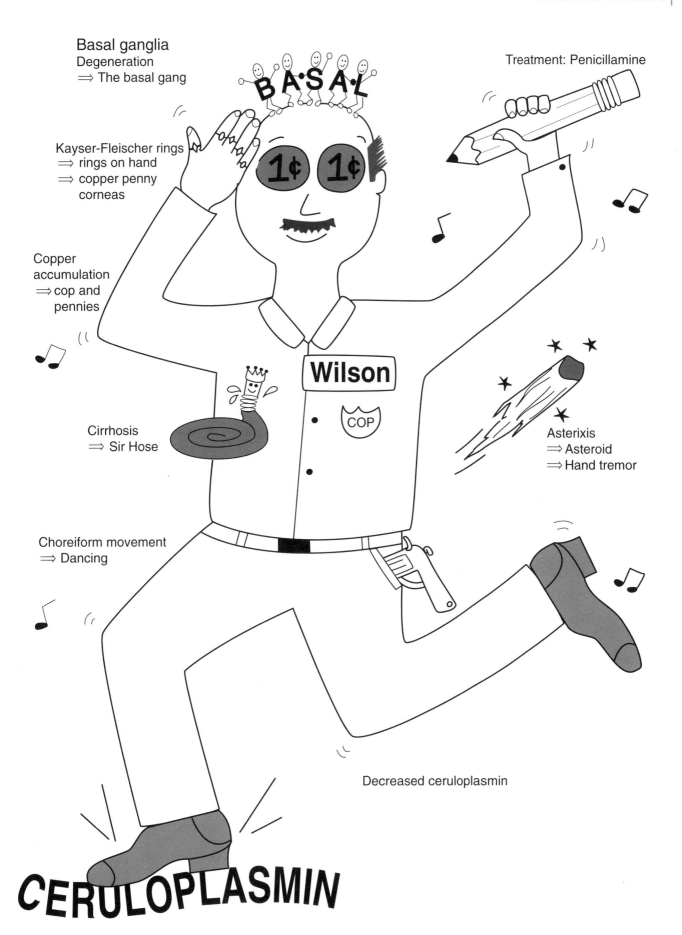

CERULOPLASMIN

NOTES

HEMOCHROMATOSIS

⇒ hero crow
- increased iron deposition results from a decrease in intestinal absorption of iron
⇒ lifting iron
- the classic triad includes
  - micronodular pigment cirrhosis
  ⇒ Sir Hose
  - skin pigmentation due to hemosiderin pigmentation ⇒ pig; hemosiderin ⇒ Sid the pig
  - diabetes mellitus ("Bronze" diabetes) bronze ⇒ 3rd place; diabetes ⇒ diet of beets
- also associated with
  - increased ferritin
  ⇒ ferret
  - reduction in total iron-binding capacity (TIBC)
  - congestive heart failure (CHF) and an increased risk of hepatocellular carcinoma
- treatment includes deferoxamine
⇒ deaf ear ox

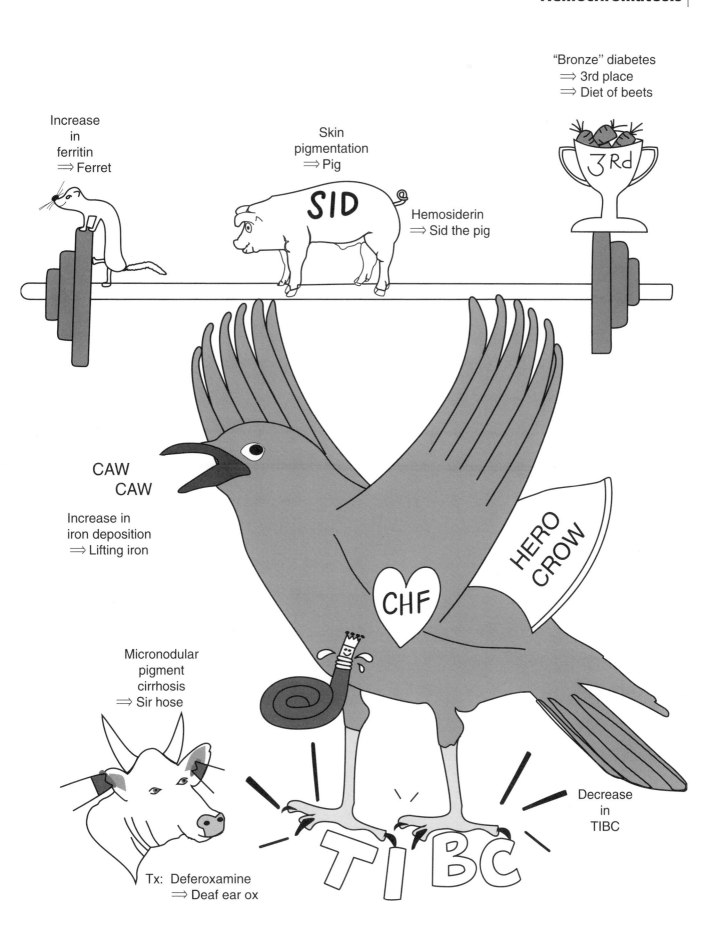

"Bronze" diabetes
⇒ 3rd place
⇒ Diet of beets

Increase
in
ferritin
⇒ Ferret

Skin
pigmentation
⇒ Pig

SID

Hemosiderin
⇒ Sid the pig

3Rd

CAW
CAW

Increase in
iron deposition
⇒ Lifting iron

HERO
CROW

CHF

Micronodular
pigment
cirrhosis
⇒ Sir hose

Decrease
in
TIBC

TIBC

Tx: Deferoxamine
⇒ Deaf ear ox

NOTES

GALLSTONES (CHOLELITHIASIS)

⇒ seagull dropping stones
- risk factors include "fat fertile females over forty"
  Fertile⇒babies; 40⇒birthday cake
- cholesterol stones
  - ⇒ butter
  - also associated with Native Americans, oral contraceptives, and Crohn's disease
    Native Americans⇒feather; Crohn's disease⇒crown
    oral contraceptives⇒pill pack
- pigment stones
  - ⇒ pig
  - composed of insoluble unconjugated bilirubin
    - ⇒ "belly rubbin'"
  - associated with hemolytic anemia, alcoholic cirrhosis, and biliary bacterial infection
    hemolytic anemia⇒lysed red blood cells (RBCs); infection and cirrhosis⇒Band-Aid and beer
- mixed stones
  - most common type of gallstone
  - composed of cholesterol and calcium salts
    - ⇒ butter and milk
- patients may present with Charcot's triad: right upper quadrant (RUQ) pain, fever, and jaundice
  fever⇒thermometer; jaundice⇒dice
- patients may also complain of fatty food intolerance

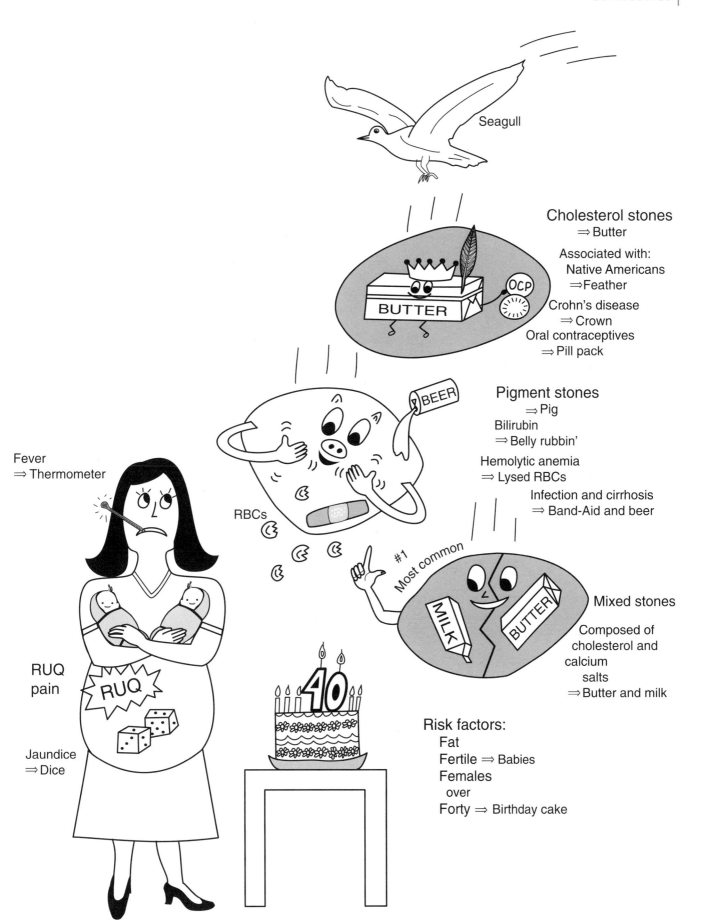

Seagull

Cholesterol stones
⇒ Butter

Associated with:
Native Americans
⇒ Feather

Crohn's disease
⇒ Crown

Oral contraceptives
⇒ Pill pack

BUTTER

OCP

Pigment stones
⇒ Pig

Bilirubin
⇒ Belly rubbin'

Hemolytic anemia
⇒ Lysed RBCs

Infection and cirrhosis
⇒ Band-Aid and beer

BEER

RBCs

Fever
⇒ Thermometer

#1 Most common

Mixed stones

MILK   BUTTER

Composed of
cholesterol and
calcium
salts
⇒ Butter and milk

RUQ
pain

RUQ

40

Risk factors:
Fat
Fertile ⇒ Babies
Females
 over
Forty ⇒ Birthday cake

Jaundice
⇒ Dice

NOTES

ACUTE PANCREATITIS

⇒ Amy's cute pants are tight
- most commonly caused by gallstones and excessive alcohol use gallstones
⇒ sea gull dropping stones
- other causes include hyperlipidemia, trauma, drugs
- pancreatic enzymes are activated and lead to the autodigestion of the pancreas
⇒ bite out of pants
- hemorrhagic fat necrosis occurs
⇒ melting butter
- calcium soap deposits lead to hypocalcemia
  calcium soap deposits⇒milk and butter; hypocalcemia⇒milk pouring
- pseudocyst formation may occur
- patients present with epigastric abdominal pain radiating to the back
- associated with elevated serum amylase, lipase, white blood cells lipase⇒lips
- Cullen's sign: periumbilical ecchymoses due to hemorrhage
⇒ periumbilical discoloration
- Grey Turner's sign: flank ecchymoses due to hemorrhage
⇒ flank discoloration

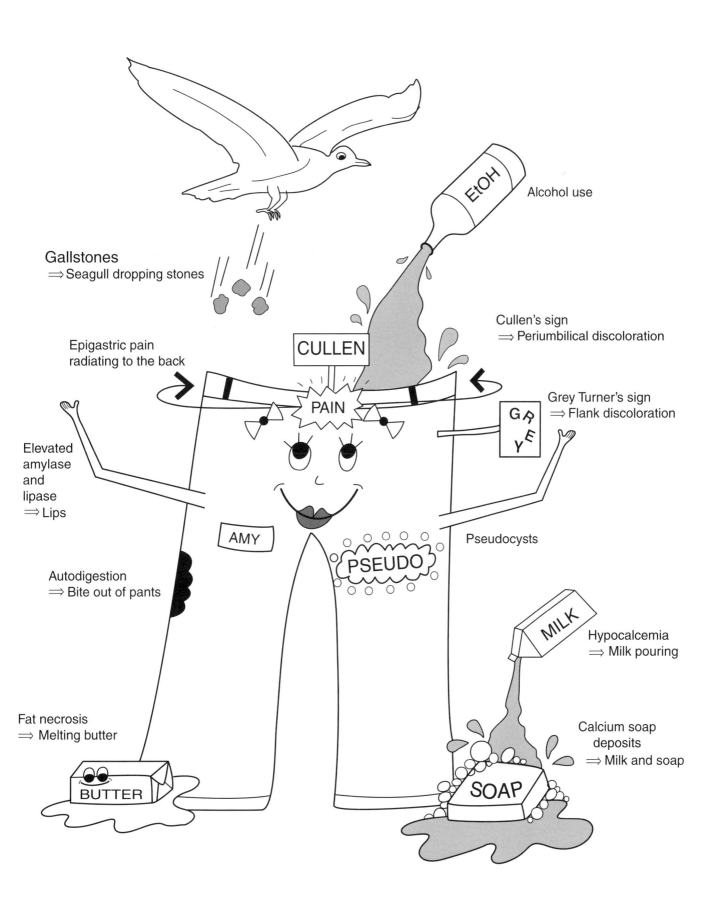

Gallstones
⟹ Seagull dropping stones

Alcohol use

Cullen's sign
⟹ Periumbilical discoloration

Epigastric pain
radiating to the back

CULLEN

PAIN

Grey Turner's sign
⟹ Flank discoloration

GREY

Elevated
amylase
and
lipase
⟹ Lips

AMY

Pseudocysts

PSEUDO

Autodigestion
⟹ Bite out of pants

Hypocalcemia
⟹ Milk pouring

MILK

Fat necrosis
⟹ Melting butter

Calcium soap
deposits
⟹ Milk and soap

BUTTER

SOAP

EtOH

NOTES

CARCINOMA OF THE PANCREAS

⇒ can of CANCER in the pan
- usually adenocarcinoma
⇒ "ADD IN NO CANCER"
- more common in smokers
- occurs most commonly in the pancreatic head leading to obstructive jaundice
⇒ head on can
- patients often present with
    - abdominal pain radiating to the back
    - weight loss and anorexia
    - migratory thrombophlebitis (Trousseau's sign)
    ⇒ trousers
    - obstructive jaundice
    - palpable gallbladder (Courvoisier's sign)
    ⇒ hand on seagull
    - pruritus
    ⇒ itching
- associated with an increase in direct bilirubin, alkaline phosphatase, and carcinoembryonic antigen (CEA)
        bilirubin⇒"belly rubbin'," rockets taking off
- poor prognosis, usually results in death within 1 year

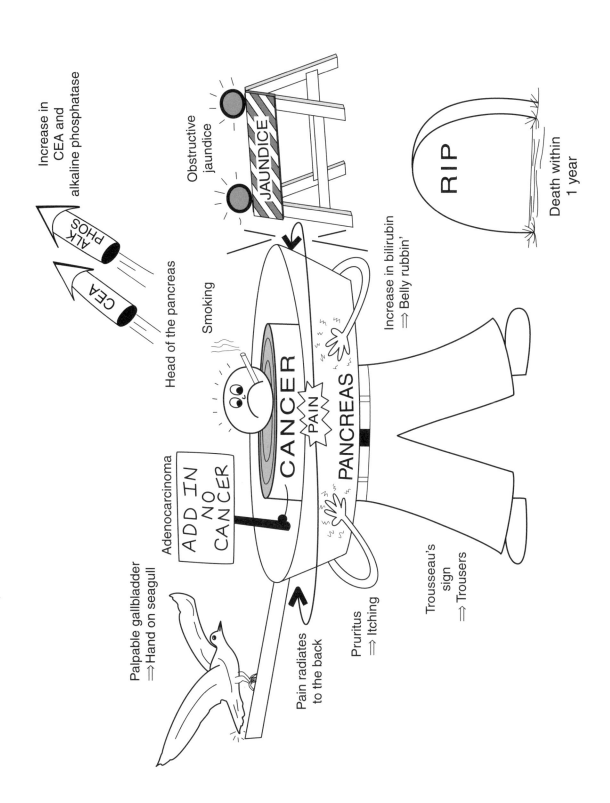

Increase in CEA and alkaline phosphatase

Obstructive jaundice

JAUNDICE

ALK PHOS

CEA

Head of the pancreas

Smoking

Increase in bilirubin
⇒ 'Belly rubbin'

RIP

Death within 1 year

Adenocarcinoma

ADD IN NO CANCER

CANCER

PAIN

PANCREAS

Palpable gallbladder
⇒ Hand on seagull

Pain radiates to the back

Pruritus
⇒ Itching

Trousseau's sign
⇒ Trousers

7.
ENDOCRINE SYSTEM

NOTES

MULTIPLE ENDOCRINE NEOPLASIA SYNDROMES (MEN SYNDROMES)

⇒ multiple men
- associated with hyperplasias or neoplasms of several endocrine organs
- autosomal dominant

MEN I

⇒ one man juggling 3 P's
- Wermer's syndrome⇒worm
- involves parathyroids, pancreas, and pituitary⇒3 P's
  - most common manifestation is hyperparathyroidism
- associated with mutation of chromosome 11

MEN II

- MEN IIA⇒two men in shape of A
  - Sipple's syndrome⇒"sippin'"
  - characterized by pheochromocytoma⇒Perry Como's sore toe; medullary carcinoma⇒muddy Larry; parathyroid hyperplasia⇒pair of thigh voids
  - thyroid medullary carcinomas occur in 100% of patients; carcinomas are foci of C-cell hyperplasia that secrete calcitonin
  - associated with chromosome 10 mutation of RET prito-oncogen
- MEN IIB (MEN III)⇒two men in shape of B, and sometimes three
  - involves medullary carcinomas, pheochromocytomas, and neuromas of skin, eyes, mouth, gastrointestinal, and respiratory tract
- familial medullary thyroid cancer⇒family of muddy Larrys in shape of A
  - variant of MEN IIA

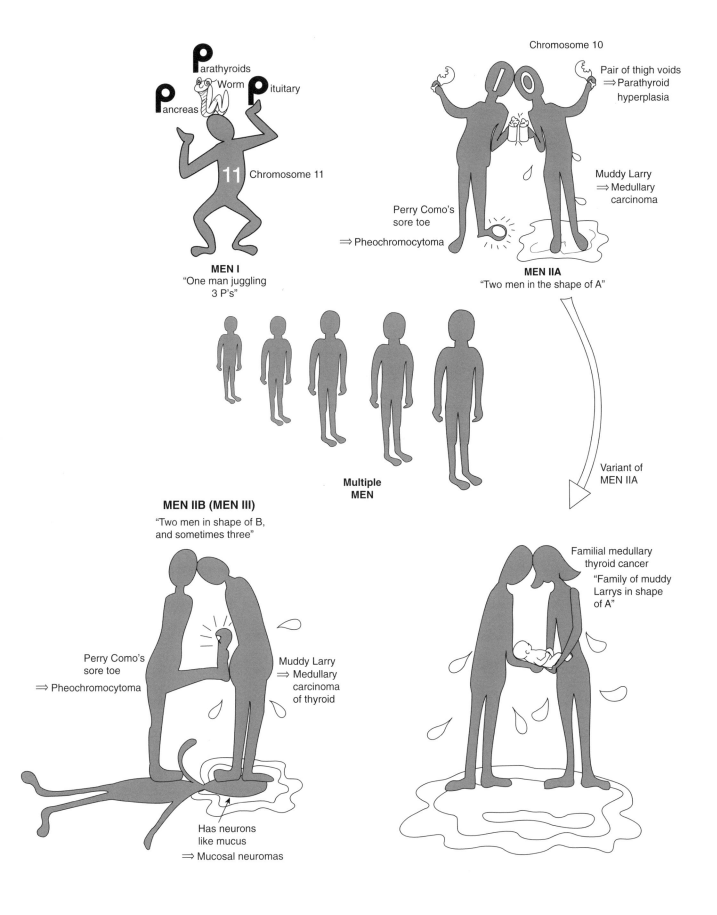

Parathyroids
Worm
Pituitary
Pancreas

Chromosome 11

11

MEN I
"One man juggling
3 P's"

Chromosome 10

Pair of thigh voids
⇒ Parathyroid
hyperplasia

Muddy Larry
⇒ Medullary
carcinoma

Perry Como's
sore toe

⇒ Pheochromocytoma

MEN IIA
"Two men in the shape of A"

**Multiple
MEN**

Variant of
MEN IIA

MEN IIB (MEN III)

"Two men in shape of B,
and sometimes three"

Perry Como's
sore toe

⇒ Pheochromocytoma

Muddy Larry
⇒ Medullary
carcinoma
of thyroid

Has neurons
like mucus
⇒ Mucosal neuromas

Familial medullary
thyroid cancer

"Family of muddy
Larrys in shape
of A"

PITUITARY GLAND

- composed of two lobes: anterior (adenohypophysis) and posterior (neurohypophysis)
- anterior pituitary: derived from Rathke's pouch (extension of oral cavity); produces the following hormones: somatotrophs (growth hormone), lactotrophs (produce prolactin), corticotrophs (adrenocorticotropic hormone [ACTH], pro-opiomelanocortin, melanocyte-stimulating hormone [MSH], endorphins, and lipotropin), thyrotrophs (thyroid-stimulating hormone [TSH]), and gonadotrophs (follicle-stimulating hormone [FSH], luteinizing hormone [LSH]).
- posterior pituitary: consists of modified glial cells (pituicytes) and axonal processes from hypothalamic nuclei (supraoptic and paraventricular); produce oxytocin and vasopressin; hormones released directly into systemic circulation

Hyperpituitarism and Pituitary Adenomas

- anterior pituitary hormone production most often caused by anterior lobe adenoma; other causes→primary hypothalamic disorders and anterior pituitary carcinomas
- adenomas can be functional (produce hormone or hormones) or nonfunctional and cause hypopituitarism by encroaching on surrounding pituitary tissue
- adenomas are usually monoclonal in origin
- morphology: adenomas are divided into macroadenomas (>1 cm diameter) and microadenomas (<1 cm diameter)
- pituitary apoplexy→acute hemorrhage into adenoma with symptoms of rapidly enlarging intracranial lesion

Present as endocrine abnormalities and mass effects; radiographic abnormalities of sella turcica; visual field abnormalities (due to close proximity of optic nerve fibers) classically present as bitemporal hemianopsia; increased intracranial pressure symptoms; or compression of adjacent nonneoplastic tissue that may result in hypopituitarism

Prolactinoma

- most frequent hyperfunctioning pituitary adenoma (30% of pituitary adenomas)
- symptoms: amenorrhea, galactorrhea, libido loss, and infertility
- other causes of hyperprolactinemia→ lactotroph hyperplasia (occurs when there is interference with dopamine inhibition of prolactin secretion), which can be due to head trauma (causing pituitary stalk section) or antidopaminergic drugs; stalk effect→mass in adjacent area interferes with hypothalamic inhibition of prolactin by protruding into stalk

- prolactinomas are treated with bromocriptine

Growth Hormone (GH) Adenoma

- GH hypersecretion causes hepatic secretion of insulin-like growth factor–I (IGF-I), which results in many symptoms; in children before the epiphyses have closed, increased GH levels result in gigantism (increase in body size, especially in arm and legs); in adults after epiphyses have closed, increased GH results in acromegaly (growth in soft tissues, skin, viscera→ thyroid, heart, liver, and adrenals), acromegaly of bones of face, hands, and feet; bone density increased in spine and hips; jaw is enlarged and protruding (prognathism); hands and feet are enlarged with broad, sausage-like fingers

Corticotroph Cell Adenoma

- corticotroph adenoma production of excess ACTH results in adrenal hypersecretion of cortisol, known as *Cushing's syndrome* (hypercortisolism)
- Cushing's disease→hypercortisolism caused by excess excretion of ACTH by pituitary

Hypopituitarism

- decreased secretion of pituitary hormones, most often from destructive processes (tumors of anterior pituitary, ischemia, empty sella syndrome)
- other causes include pituitary surgery or radiation; genetic defects; Rathke's cleft cyst; pituitary apoplexy (with sudden onset of extremely painful headache, diplopia, and hypopituitarism); Sheehan's syndrome (postpartum necrosis of anterior pituitary)
- empty sella syndrome→any condition that destroys part or all of pituitary gland
- presents with hypothyroidism, hypoadrenalism, pallor, amenorrhea, impotence, loss of libido, loss of pubic and axillary hair

Posterior Pituitary Syndromes

- posterior pituitary secretes oxytocin and vasopressin (antidiuretic hormone [ADH])
- oxytocin stimulates uterine smooth muscle and cells surrounding lactiferous ducts of mammary glands; excess oxytocin release has not been implicated with clinical significance
- ADH excess production causes clinical syndromes, including diabetes insipidus and secretion of inappropriately high levels of ADH (SIADH)
- diabetes insipidus: ADH deficiency causes excessive urination as a result of the kidney's inability to resorb water from urine, which leads to large amounts of dilute urine and increased serum

sodium and osmolality, in turn resulting in thirst and polydipsia
- syndrome of inappropriate ADH (SIADH): ADH excess causes resorption of excessive amounts of free water, resulting in hyponatremia; most frequent causes include the secretion of ectopic ADH by malignant neoplasms (especially small cell carcinoma of the lung); clinical manifestations→ hyponatremia, cerebral edema, and neurologic dysfunction; total body water is increased, blood volume remains normal→therefore, peripheral edema does not develop

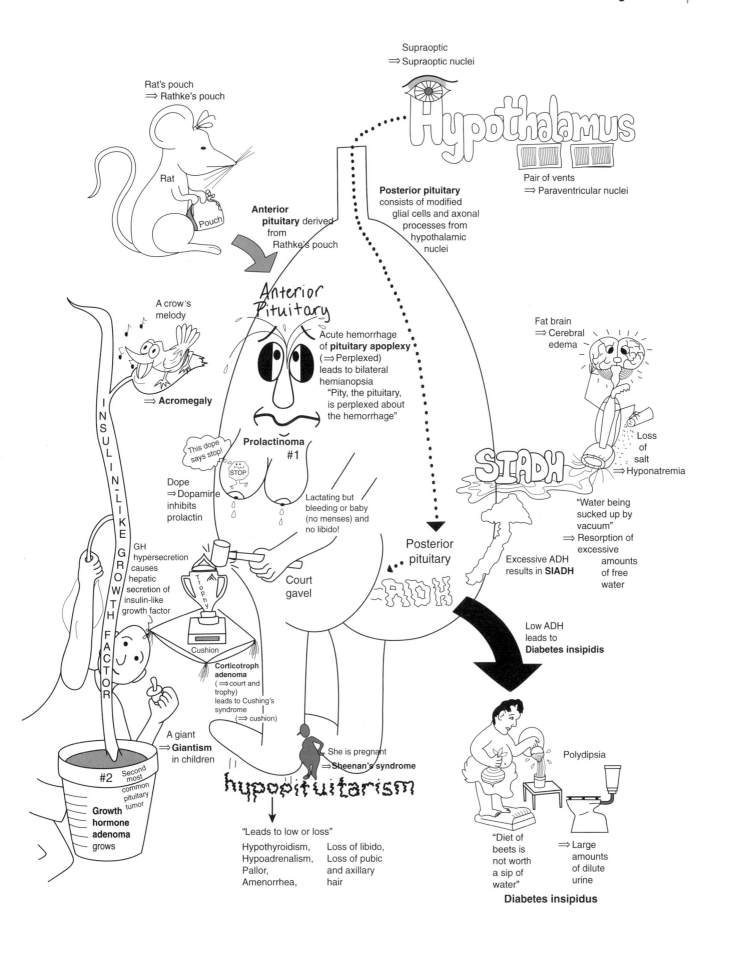

Supraoptic
⇒ Supraoptic nuclei

Rat's pouch
⇒ Rathke's pouch

Rat

Pouch

Anterior pituitary derived from Rathke's pouch

Posterior pituitary consists of modified glial cells and axonal processes from hypothalamic nuclei

Pair of vents
⇒ Paraventricular nuclei

A crow's melody

⇒ **Acromegaly**

Anterior Pituitary

Acute hemorrhage of **pituitary apoplexy** (⇒ Perplexed) leads to bilateral hemianopsia
"Pity, the pituitary, is perplexed about the hemorrhage"

Fat brain
⇒ Cerebral edema

Prolactinoma #1

This dope says stop!

STOP

Dope
⇒ Dopamine inhibits prolactin

Lactating but bleeding or baby (no menses) and no libido!

Loss of salt
⇒ Hyponatremia

"Water being sucked up by vacuum"
⇒ Resorption of excessive amounts of free water

Excessive ADH results in **SIADH**

GH hypersecretion causes hepatic secretion of insulin-like growth factor

Trophy

Cushion

Posterior pituitary

ADH

Low ADH leads to **Diabetes insipidis**

I
N
S
U
L
I
N
-
L
I
K
E
G
R
O
W
T
H
F
A
C
T
O
R

Court gavel

Corticotroph adenoma (⇒ court and trophy) leads to Cushing's syndrome (⇒ cushion)

A giant
⇒ **Giantism** in children

She is pregnant
Sheenan's syndrome

hypopituitarism

Polydipsia

#2 Second most common pituitary tumor

Growth hormone adenoma grows

"Leads to low or loss"

Hypothyroidism,
Hypoadrenalism,
Pallor,
Amenorrhea,

Loss of libido,
Loss of pubic and axillary hair

"Diet of beets is not worth a sip of water"

⇒ Large amounts of dilute urine

Diabetes insipidus

PARATHYROID

- derived from developing pharyngeal pouches that also give rise to thymus
- lies in close proximity to the upper and lower poles of each thyroid lobe
- mostly composed of chief cells that contain secretory granules of parathyroid hormone (PTH); also contains oxyphil cells
- activity controlled by level of free (ionized) calcium in blood; decreased calcium stimulates synthesis and secretion of PTH
- metabolic functions of PTH: activates osteoclasts; increases the renal tubular reabsorption of calcium; increases the conversion of vitamin D to its active dihydroxy form in the kidneys (this form of vitamin D is important for calcium transport across the gastrointestinal tract); increases urinary phosphate excretion; augments gastrointestinal calcium absorption
- hypercalcemia→result of elevated levels of PTH and malignancy
- hypercalcemia due to malignancy occurs because of osteolytic metastases and local release of cytokines (which induce local osteolysis) and release of PTH-related protein (binds to PTH receptors and causes same reactions as PTH would)

Hyperparathyroidism

- primary (due to autonomous PTH overproduction); secondary and tertiary (due to chronic renal insufficiency)
- **primary**→caused by adenoma, primary hyperplasia, and parathyroid carcinoma
- commoner in women in their 50s or later; patients have a history of irradiation 30 to 40 years before onset
- clinically may be asymptomatic (only manifestation is increased serum ionized calcium level) or symptomatic (painful bones, renal stones, abdominal groans, and psychic moans)
- patients with primary hyperparathyroidism have an increased serum PTH level, whereas PTH levels are low in hypercalcemia caused by nonparathyroid disease
- **secondary**→renal failure commonest cause; other causes include inadequate intake of calcium, steatorrhea, and vitamin D deficiency
- renal insufficiency also decreases phosphate excretion, resulting in hyperphosphatemia, which further depresses serum calcium levels (formation of calcium phosphate) and by doing so stimulates parathyroid activity

Hypoparathyroidism

- deficient PTH
- causes: surgical removal; congenital absence of all glands; idiopathic atrophy; familial (associated with candidiasis and adrenal insufficiency)
- clinically presents with tetany; neuromuscular irritability (with positive Chvostek's sign→tapping of facial nerve induces facial contractions of eye, nose, and mouth; and positive Trousseau's sign→occluding forearm circulation induces carpal spasm, which disappears when occlusion taken away)
- mental status changes; ocular disease (calcification of lens); cardiovascular (prolonged QT interval)

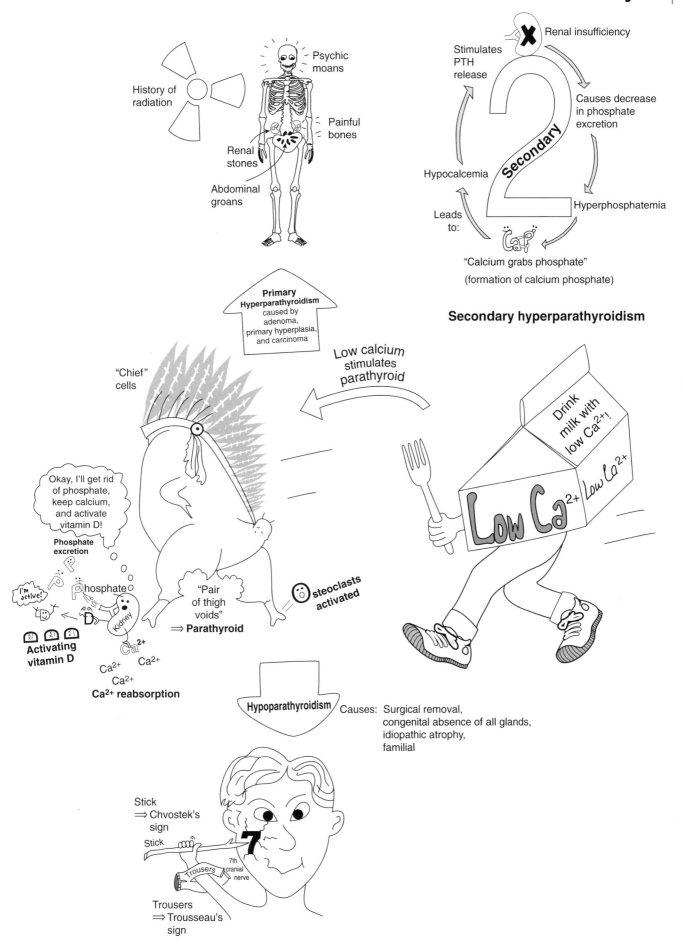

History of radiation

Psychic moans

Painful bones

Renal stones

Abdominal groans

Renal insufficiency

Stimulates PTH release

Causes decrease in phosphate excretion

Secondary

Hypocalcemia

Hyperphosphatemia

Leads to:

"Calcium grabs phosphate"
(formation of calcium phosphate)

Secondary hyperparathyroidism

Primary Hyperparathyroidism
caused by adenoma, primary hyperplasia, and carcinoma

Low calcium stimulates parathyroid

"Chief" cells

Okay, I'll get rid of phosphate, keep calcium, and activate vitamin D!

Phosphate excretion

I'm active!

Phosphate

D

Kidney

Activating vitamin D

Ca^{2+}
Ca^{2+} Ca^{2+}
Ca^{2+}

Ca^{2+} reabsorption

"Pair of thigh voids"
⇒ **Parathyroid**

steoclasts activated

Drink milk with low Ca^{2+}!

Low Ca^{2+} Low Ca^{2+}

Hypoparathyroidism Causes: Surgical removal, congenital absence of all glands, idiopathic atrophy, familial

Stick ⇒ Chvostek's sign

Stick

7th cranial nerve

Trousers

Trousers ⇒ Trousseau's sign

NOTES

THYROID

- develops from evagination of developing pharyngeal epithelium and then descends to anterior neck position
- TSH causes follicular epithelial cells to pinocytize colloid and convert thyroglobulin into thyroxine (T4) and tri-iodothyronine (T3)
- T3 and T4 are released into the systemic circulation and transported by plasma proteins to peripheral tissues, where the net effect is increased basal metabolic rate
- goitrogens→inhibit thyroid function by suppressing T3 and T4 synthesis; this, in turn, causes an increase in TSH→the increased amounts of TSH cause hyperplastic gland enlargement or goiter
  - large amounts of iodide inhibit thyroid hormone release when the patient has a hyperactive thyroid
- parafollicular cells (C cells)→synthesize and secrete calcitonin, which increases bone absorption of calcium and decreases osteoclast bone resorption

Hyperthyroidism

- elevated T3 and T4 levels (thyrotoxicosis when due to excessive leakage of hormone from a nonhyperfunctioning gland and known as *hyperthyroidism* when due to hyperfunctioning thyroid)
- physical manifestations→nervousness, palpitations, heat intolerance, weight loss even with good appetite, excessive perspiration, osteoporosis, warm moist and flushed skin, overactivity of sympathetic nervous system, diarrhea, and ocular changes
- causes→diffuse hyperplasia, exogenous thyroid hormone, thyroiditis, hyperfunctioning multinodular goiter or adenoma
- diagnosis→TSH and unbound T4 measurement (a low TSH and high T4 would indicate primary hyperthyroidism due to intrinsic thyroid disease, not thyrotoxicosis caused by hypothalamic or pituitary disease, also known as *secondary hyperthyroidism*)
- thyrotropin releasing hormone (TRH) stimulation test→determination of primary versus secondary→a rise in TSH after a TRH injection excludes secondary hyperthyroidism
- T3 hyperthyroidism→high serum T3, low TSH, and normal T4→due to increased T3 secretion and peripheral conversion of T4 to T3
- treatment→β-blockers, thionamide, iodine, inhibitors of T4 to T3 conversion, and radioiodine

Hypothyroidism

- low levels of thyroid hormone
- primary hypothyroidism→most common cause in iodine-sufficient areas is chronic autoimmune thyroiditits or Hashimoto's thyroiditis; other causes→radiation, drugs, surgery
- secondary hypothyroidism→TSH deficiency and tertiary hypothyroidism are caused by TRH deficiency
- clinical→cretinism and myxedema
- cretinism: hypothyroidism in childhood or infancy; clinical manifestations: severe mental retardation, short stature, coarse facial features, protruding tongue, and umbilical hernia
- Myxedema: hypothyroidism in child or adult; slowing of physical and mental activity, including fatigue, apathy, cold intolerance, overweight, reduced cardiac output, shortness of breath, decreased exercise capacity, constipation, decreased sweating, and cool and pale skin
- TSH increases in patients with intrinsic thyroid disease because of the loss of T4 and T3 feedback inhibition on pituitary TSH production
- TSH is not increased in patients with hypothalamic or pituitary disease
- in all cases T4 is decreased

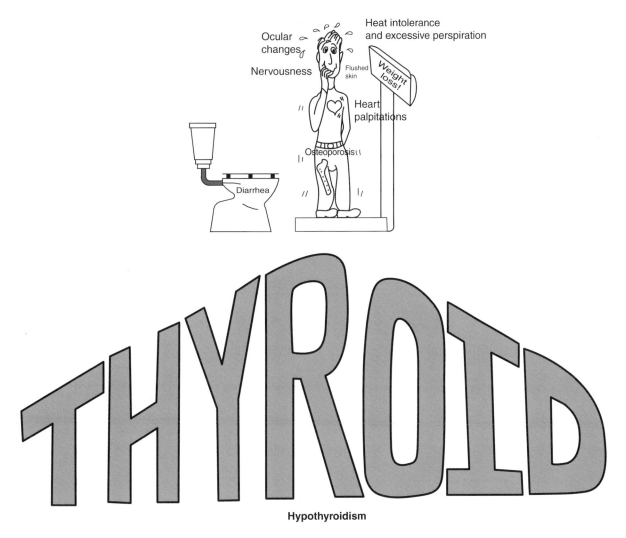

Hypothyroidism

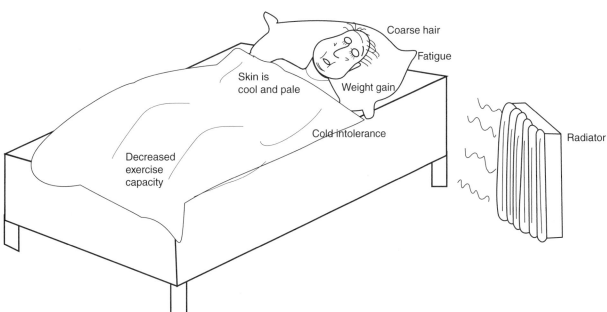

NOTES

GRAVES' DISEASE

- most common cause of endogenous hyperthyroidism
- triad of findings: hyperthyroidism, infiltrative ophthalmopathy (exophthalmos), localized infiltrative dermopathy (pretibial myxedema)
- common in women between ages 20 and 40; associated with human leukocyte antigen (HLA) B8 and DR3
- autoimmune disorder with autoantibodies to TSH receptor that is specific for Graves' disease
- ophthalmopathy→retro-orbital connective tissue and extraocular muscles' volume increased due to inflammation
- morphology: symmetrically enlarged; diffuse hypertrophy and hyperplasia; histologically, there are too many cells; follicular epithelial cells tall and crowded; crowding results in papillae that project into lumen and encroach on the colloid; colloid is pale with scalloped margins
- clinical: diffuse thyroid enlargement; audible bruit due to increased flow of blood through hyperactive gland; ophthalmopathy; wide staring gaze and lid lag; exophthalmos; pretibial myxedema (scaly thickening and induration of skin over shins)
- radioactive iodine uptake is increased

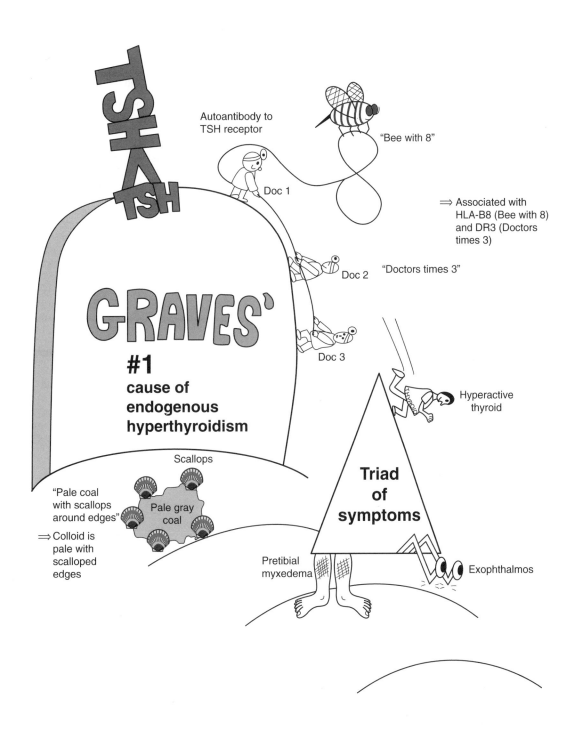

Autoantibody to
TSH receptor

"Bee with 8"

Doc 1

Doc 2

"Doctors times 3"

Doc 3

⇒ Associated with
HLA-B8 (Bee with 8)
and DR3 (Doctors
times 3)

GRAVES'

#1
**cause of
endogenous
hyperthyroidism**

Hyperactive
thyroid

Scallops

"Pale coal
with scallops
around edges"

Pale gray
coal

⇒ Colloid is
pale with
scalloped
edges

**Triad
of
symptoms**

Pretibial
myxedema

Exophthalmos

NOTES

THYROID NEOPLASMS

- 90% of neoplastic nodules are adenomas
- neoplastic nodules→solitary in younger patients, more common in males, history of radiation, most likely do not take up radioiodine

Adenomas

- derived from follicular adenomas
- pathogenesis: somatic mutations cause chronic stimulation of cyclic adenosine monophosphate (cAMP) pathway of TSH receptor→creating cells that continually grow
- histologic subtypes: colloid adenomas (large colloid-filled follicles); fetal adenomas (numerous small follicles separated by loose myxoid stroma); trabecular adenomas (closely packed cells forming cords with few follicles); atypical adenomas or spindle cell adenomas; Hürthle-cell adenoma; papillary adenoma
- clinical: painless mass; take up less radioiodine than normal thyroid
- carcinomas arise *de novo* and not from transformation of adenoma

Carcinomas

- uncommon in United States
- more common in women in early to middle adult years
- estrogen receptor expression on neoplasm
- subtypes: papillary, follicular, medullary, anaplastic
- major risk factor: previous exposure to ionizing radiation, especially during first 20 years; other predisposing factors include nodular goiter and Hashimoto's thyroiditis
- causes: activation or mutation of oncogenes (RET proto-oncogene on chromosome 10→papillary and medullary thyroid cancers)

Papillary Carcinoma

- most common type of thyroid cancer; higher incidence in patients with Gardner's syndrome and Cowden's disease
- microscopic examination: branching papillae with fibrovascular stalk covered by cuboidal epithelial cells; Orphan Annie nuclei (finely dispersed chromatin); eosinophilic intranuclear inclusions; psammoma bodies (calcified lesions)→**DIAGNOSTIC OF PAPILLARY CARCINOMA**
- clinical: asymptomatic thyroid nodules; mass in cervical lymph nodes; moves freely during swallowing; advanced disease→dysphagia, cough, or dyspnea
- cold lesions on scintiscans

Follicular Carcinoma

- second most common thyroid cancer; more common in older women (40s and 50s); increased in iodine-deficient areas; single nodules; nuclei lack papillary carcinoma features, and psammoma bodies are not present
- clinical: slowly enlarging painless nodules; cold nodules on scintigrams; lymph nodes rarely involved; vascular invasion common; treated with lobectomy or subtotal thyroidectomy

Medullary Carcinoma

- neuroendocrine neoplasm derived from parafollicular cells (C cells); secrete calcitonin and other hormones→ carcinoembryonic antigen (CEA), somatostatin, serotonin, and vasoactive intestinal peptide (VIP)
- 80% arise sporadically and rest associated with MEN IIA and IIB or familial tumors
- morphology: familial cases→multiple foci of C-cell hyperplasia
- clinical: sporadic cases→ paraneoplastic syndrome usually manifests first (e.g., diarrhea due to VIP secretion from neoplasm); familial cases→usually asymptomatic and discovered through screening relatives of patients with the carcinoma

Anaplastic Carcinoma

- undifferentiated tumors of thyroid follicular epithelium; aggressive→ mortality near 100%
- clinical: present as rapidly enlarging bulky neck mass and usually metastasized when diagnosed; no effective therapy

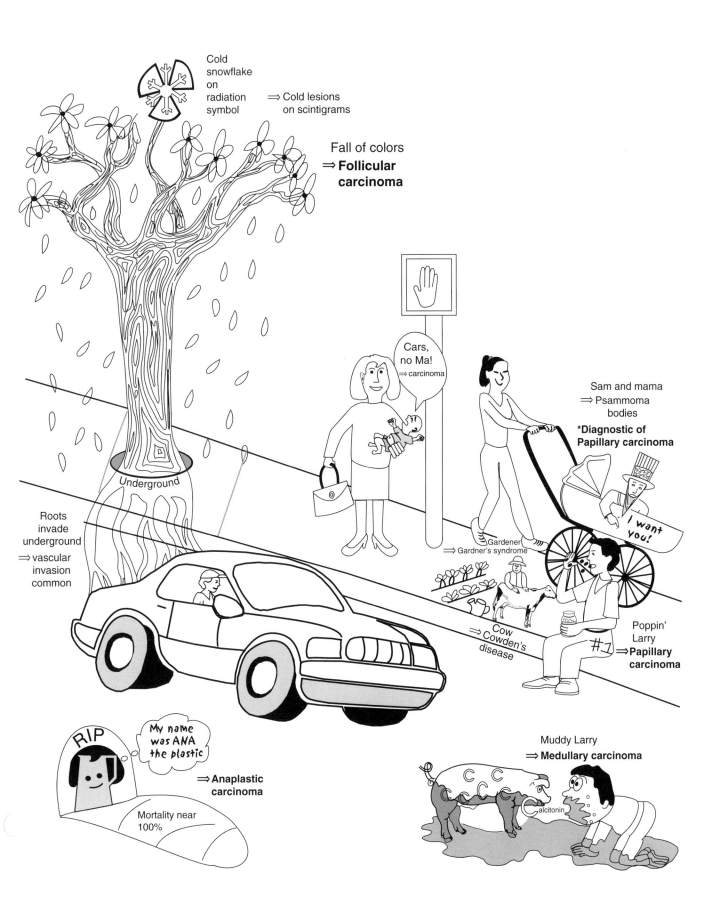

THYROIDITIS

- inflammation of thyroid
- sudden onset of neck pain, tenderness in neck, fever, chills
- types→Hashimoto's; subacute granulomatous; subacute lymphocytic

Hashimoto's Thyroiditis

- most common cause of hypothyroidism in iodine-sufficient areas; gradual thyroid failure
- autoimmune destruction of gland; common in women 45 to 65 years old
- clusters in families; associated with HLA DR5 and DR3
- transient hyperthyroidism may occur when inflammation causes disruption of thyroid follicular cells
- associated with increased incidence of other autoimmune diseases including systemic lupus erythematosus (SLE) and rheumatoid arthritis
- caused by defect in T cells; B-lymphocytes secrete autoantibodies directed against thyroid antigens (thyroglobulin and thyroid peroxidase)
- autoantibodies can fix complement
- morphology: diffusely enlarged thyroid; thyroid follicles small and lined by epithelial cells with eosinophilic granular cytoplasm (Hürthle cells)
- clinical: painless enlargement of thyroid; some degree of hypothyroidism that may be preceded by transient thyrotoxicosis

Subacute (Granulomatous) Thyroiditis

- also granulomatous thyroiditis or DeQuervain's thyroiditis
- caused by viral infection of postviral inflammatory process; patients have upper respiratory infection before onset; peak incidence during summer months
- morphology: multinucleate giant cells enclose colloid fragments
- clinical: pain in neck that radiates to upper neck, jaw, throat, or ears, especially when swallowing; transient hyperthyroidism followed by asymptomatic hypothyroidism

Subacute Lymphocytic (Painless) Thyroiditis

- also known as painless, silent, or lymphocytic thyroiditis; uncommon cause of hyperthyroidism
- morphology: multifocal inflammatory infiltrate composed of small lymphocytes and patchy disruption and collapse of thyroid follicles
- clinical: main symptom is hyperthyroidism that lasts 2 to 8 weeks; ophthalmopathy not present
- laboratory findings→elevated T4 and T3 with lowered TSH levels; radioactive iodine uptake is decreased

Reidel's Thyroiditis

- less common; extensive thyroid fibrosis and contiguous neck structure fibrosis; associated with idiopathic fibrosis in other body areas, for example, retroperitoneum

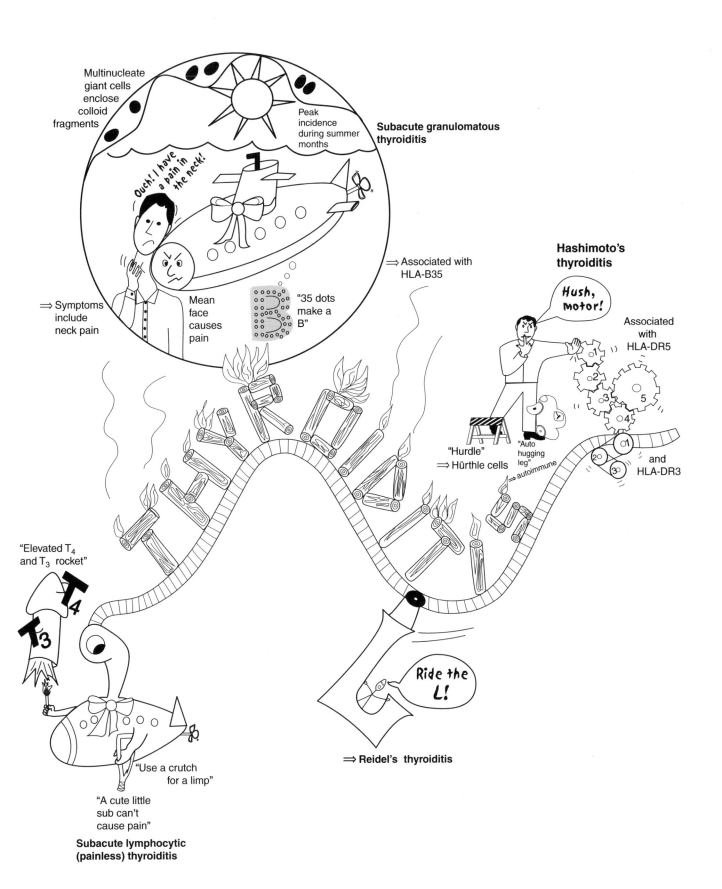

Multinucleate giant cells enclose colloid fragments

Peak incidence during summer months

Subacute granulomatous thyroiditis

"Ouch! I have a pain in the neck!"

⟹ Associated with HLA-B35

⟹ Symptoms include neck pain

Mean face causes pain

"35 dots make a B"

Hashimoto's thyroiditis

Hush, motor!

Associated with HLA-DR5

"Hurdle"
⟹ Hürthle cells

"Auto hugging leg" → autoimmune

and HLA-DR3

"Elevated T₄ and T₃ rocket"

Ride the L!

"Use a crutch for a limp"

"A cute little sub can't cause pain"

Subacute lymphocytic (painless) thyroiditis

⟹ **Reidel's thyroiditis**

NOTES

DIFFUSE AND MULTINODULAR GOITER

- most common manifestation of thyroid disease; reflects impaired thyroid hormone synthesis usually caused by iodine deficiency
- degree of enlargement relative to thyroid hormone deficiency

Diffuse Nontoxic (Simple) Goiter

- goiter of entire gland without nodules; also known as *colloid goiter*
- endemic goiter (causes goitrogens; excessive calcium and certain vegetables in *Brassica* and *Cruciferae* families→cabbage, cauliflower, Brussels sprouts, turnips, and cassava)
- sporadic goiter more common in girls in puberty and young adult life (caused by hereditary enzymatic defects that interfere with thyroid synthesis); in children may cause cretinism
- morphology: two stages→hyperplastic and colloid

Multinodular Goiter

- recurrent episodes of hyperplasia and involution
- established simple goiters can convert to multinodular goiters
- produce most extreme thyroid enlargement; enlargement pattern unpredictable; pressure on midline structures such as trachea and esophagus; goiter may grow behind sternum and clavicles→intrathoracic or plunging goiter
- clinical: mass effects of enlarged gland→airway obstruction, dysphagia, and compression of large neck and upper thorax blood vessels; patients usually euthyroid (normal thyroid gland function), but a hyperfunctioning nodule may develop resulting in hyperthyroidism (Plummer's syndrome); hyperfunctioning nodules take *of* radioiodine and appear "hot"

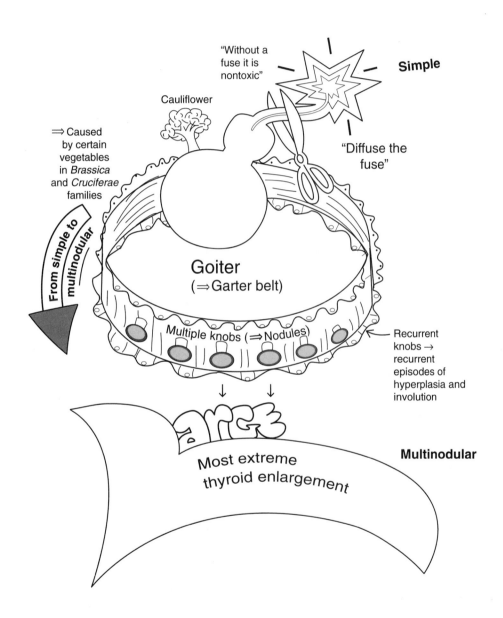

"Without a
fuse it is
nontoxic"

Simple

"Diffuse the
fuse"

Cauliflower

⇒ Caused
by certain
vegetables
in *Brassica*
and *Cruciferae*
families

From simple to
multinodular

Goiter
(⇒Garter belt)

Multiple knobs (⇒Nodules)

Recurrent
knobs →
recurrent
episodes of
hyperplasia and
involution

Most extreme
thyroid enlargement

Multinodular

NOTES

ADRENAL CORTEX

layers
- capsule
- zona glomerulosa→produces mineralocorticoids (aldosterone)
- zona fasciculata→produces glucocorticoids (cortisol)
- zona reticularis→produces androgens and glucocorticoids
- medulla→chromaffin cells produce catecholamines (epinephrine)

Hyperadrenalism

- three types: Cushing's syndrome (excess cortisol), hyperaldosteronism, adrenogenital or virilizing syndromes (excess androgens)

Adrenal Insufficiency

- types: primary acute adrenocortical insufficiency (adrenal crisis), primary chronic adrenocortical insufficiency (Addison's disease), secondary adrenocortical insufficiency

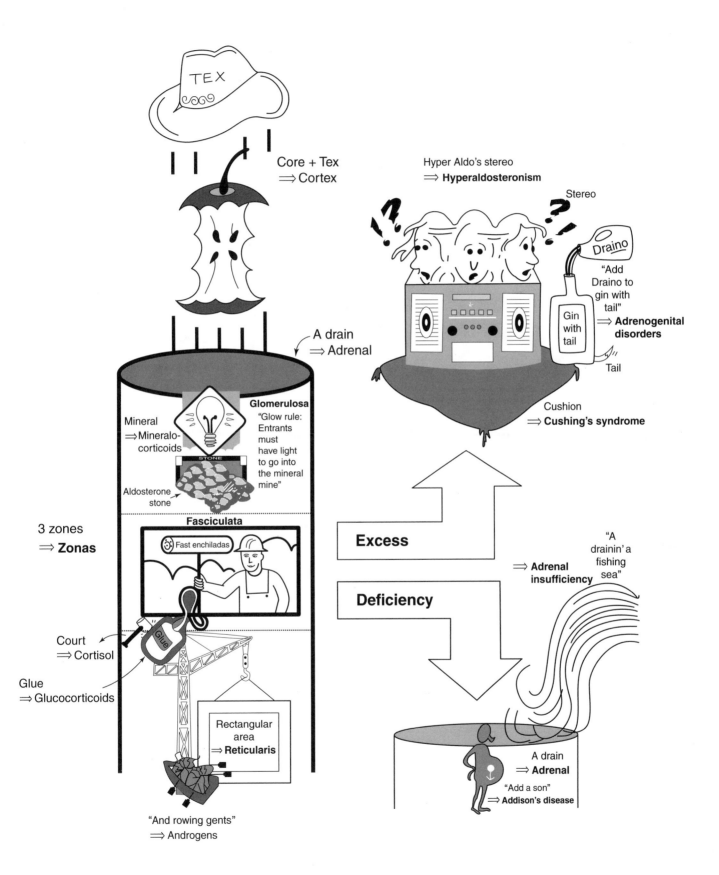

Core + Tex ⟹ Cortex

Hyper Aldo's stereo ⟹ **Hyperaldosteronism**

Stereo

Draino

"Add Draino to gin with tail" ⟹ **Adrenogenital disorders**

Gin with tail

Tail

A drain ⟹ Adrenal

Cushion ⟹ **Cushing's syndrome**

Mineral ⟹ Mineralo-corticoids

Glomerulosa
"Glow rule: Entrants must have light to go into the mineral mine"

Aldosterone stone

3 zones ⟹ **Zonas**

Fasciculata

Fast enchiladas

Excess

⟹ **Adrenal insufficiency**

"A drainin' a fishing sea"

Deficiency

Court ⟹ Cortisol

Glue ⟹ Glucocorticoids

Rectangular area ⟹ **Reticularis**

A drain ⟹ **Adrenal**

"Add a son" ⟹ **Addison's disease**

"And rowing gents" ⟹ Androgens

NOTES

CUSHING'S SYNDROME (HYPERCORTISOLISM)

- four sources of excess cortisol: most causes from intake of exogenous glucocorticoids and others associated with endogenous cortisol production from→primary hypothalamic-pituitary diseases associated with hypersecretion of ACTH; hypersecretion of cortisol by adrenal adenoma, carcinoma, or nodular hyperplasia; secretion of ectopic ACTH by nonendocrine neoplasm
- primary hypersecretion of ACTH: more common in women in 20s to 30s; most patients have small ACTH-producing adenoma in pituitary
- primary adrenal neoplasms: ACTH-independent Cushing's syndrome or adrenal Cushing's syndrome because adrenals function autonomously; with unilateral neoplasm→uninvolved adrenal cortex and opposite adrenal gland cortex undergo atrophy because of suppression of ACTH secretion; therefore, patient will have elevated cortisol levels but low levels of ACTH
- secretion of ectopic ACTH by nonpituitary tumors→most often small cell carcinoma of lung; adrenal glands undergo bilateral cortical hyperplasia
- morphology: pituitary→most common change is due to high levels of glucocorticoids and results in accumulation of keratin in cytoplasm called *Crooke's hyaline change*
- clinical: early symptoms include hypertension and weight gain; later central pattern of adipose tissue deposition (truncal obesity, moon facies, accumulation of fat in posterior neck and back)→buffalo hump; proximal muscle weakness; induction of gluconeogenesis and inhibition of glucose uptake by cells→result in hyperglycemia, glucosuria, and polydipsia; loss of collagen and bone resorption→results in thin skin and easy bruising; poor wound healing; abdominal cutaneous striae; suppression of immune response; mental disturbances; hirsutism; and menstrual abnormalities
- diagnosis: 24-hour urine where free cortisol level is increased and loss of normal diurnal pattern of cortisol secretion (normally, cortisol released in the morning and gradual reduction throughout the day; in Cushing's syndrome no reduction occurs)
- determining cause: by administration of dexamethasone and then measurement of resulting ACTH and urinary excretion of steroid→in pituitary Cushing's syndrome ACTH levels are elevated but are reduced with HIGH doses of dexamethasone, with resultant suppression of urinary steroid secretion; other causes are not affected by dexamethasone at all

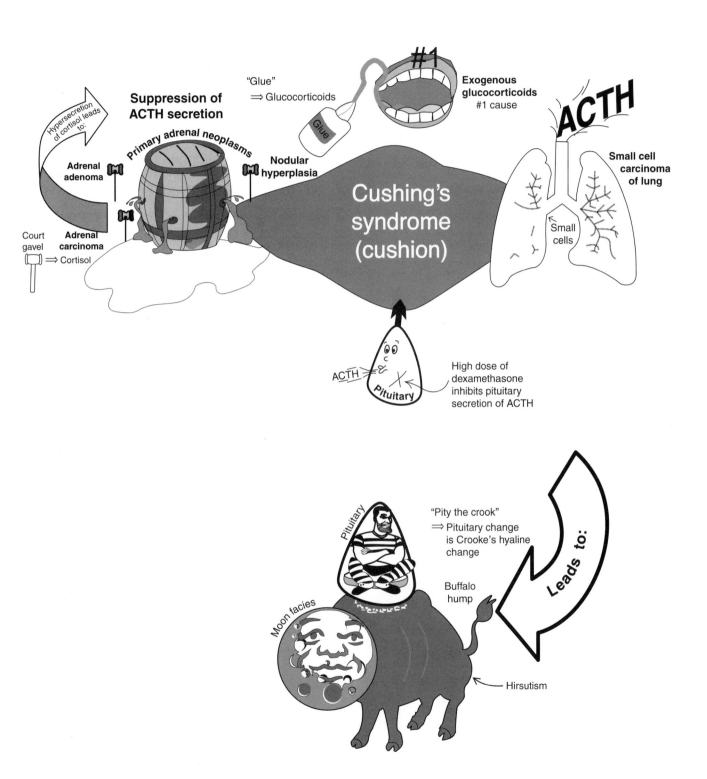

Suppression of ACTH secretion

Hypersecretion of cortisol leads to:

Primary adrenal neoplasms

Adrenal adenoma

Court gavel ⇒ Cortisol

Adrenal carcinoma

Nodular hyperplasia

"Glue" ⇒ Glucocorticoids

Glue

#1

Exogenous glucocorticoids #1 cause

ACTH

Small cell carcinoma of lung

Small cells

Cushing's syndrome (cushion)

ACTH

Pituitary

High dose of dexamethasone inhibits pituitary secretion of ACTH

Pituitary

"Pity the crook" ⇒ Pituitary change is Crooke's hyaline change

Buffalo hump

Leads to:

Moon facies

Hirsutism

NOTES

HYPERALDOSTERONISM

- chronic excess aldosterone secretion causes sodium retention (results in hypertension) and potassium excretion (results in hypokalemia)
- primary hyperaldosteronism: autonomous overproduction of aldosterone→results in suppression of renin-angiotensin system; caused by aldosterone-producing adrenocortical neoplasm or adrenocortical hyperplasia; Conn's syndrome→aldosterone-secreting adenoma in one adrenal gland that is more common in middle-aged women
- secondary hyperaldosteronism: aldosterone is released in response to renin-angiotensin system activation, which occurs in congestive heart failure, decreased renal perfusion, hypoalbuminemia, and pregnancy
- clinical: primary→hypertension, hypokalemia, low serum renin, muscle weakness, paresthesias, visual disturbances, tetany, sodium retention

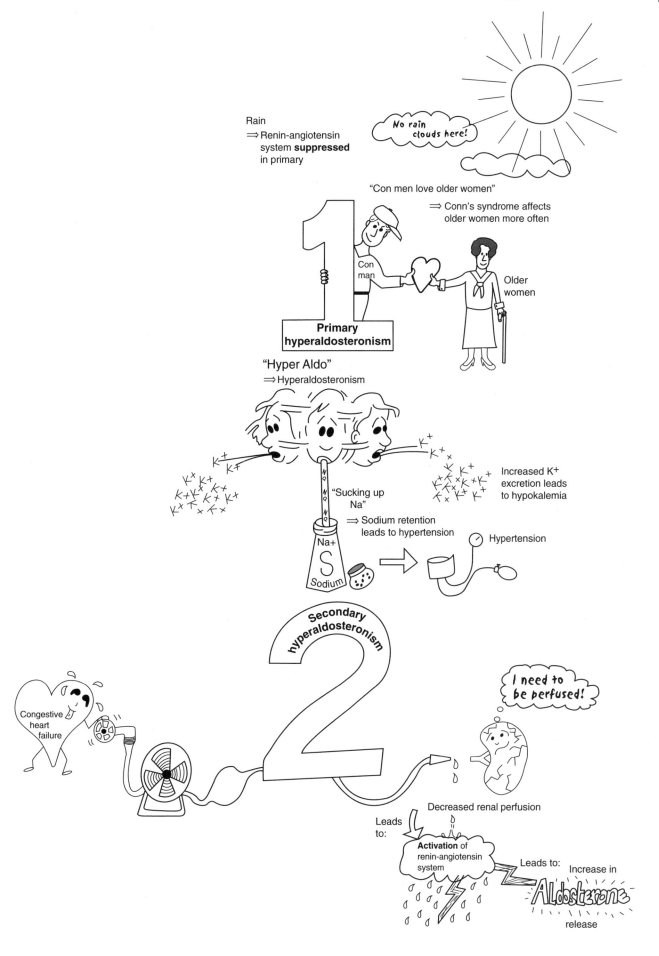

NOTES

ADRENOGENITAL SYNDROMES

- disorders of sexual differentiation (e.g., virilization); caused by gonadal disorders, adrenocortical neoplasms, and congenital adrenal hyperplasia
- adrenal neoplasms more likely to be carcinomas
- congenital adrenal hyperplasia→ autosomal recessive; inherited metabolic errors; deficiency of particular enzyme involved in biosynthesis of cortical steroids (especially cortisol); when deficiency occurs steroidogenesis is channeled to other pathways, causing increased androgen production resulting in virilization; also, there is simultaneous deficiency of cortisol, leading to increased ACTH secretion and adrenal hyperplasia

21-Hydroxylase Deficiency

- adrenal steroid synthesis: cholesterol→ pregnenolone→progesterone and 17α-hydroxyprogesterone (21-hydroxylase is needed to convert progesterone to deoxycorticosterone and also needed to convert 17α-hydroxylase to deoxycortisol)
- deficiency of 21-hydroxylase would therefore inhibit aldosterone and cortisol synthesis, which in turn causes steroid synthesis to be shifted to androgen production, resulting in three syndromes depending on the severity of mutation
  - ○ salt-wasting adrenogenitalism
  - ○ simple virilizing adrenogenitalism
  - ○ nonclassic adrenogenitalism
- salt-wasting syndrome results from total lack of hydroxylase; deficient mineralocorticoid and glucocorticoid synthesis; clinical→salt wasting, hyponatremia, hyperkalemia, which causes acidosis, hypotension, cardiovascular collapse, and possible death; excess production of androgens leads to virilization; because there is no cortisol-negative feedback to the pituitary, ACTH production is increased causing bilateral adrenal hyperplasia
- simple virilizing adrenogenital syndrome without salt wasting; less than total hydroxylase defect→enough enzyme to allow salt reabsorption, but low glucocorticoid levels are not enough for negative feedback, and ACTH is elevated with resultant adrenal hyperplasia
- nonclassic or late-onset adrenal virilism: usually asymptomatic with only mild manifestations such as hirsutism
- treatment of congenital adrenal hyperplasia→exogenous glucocorticoids

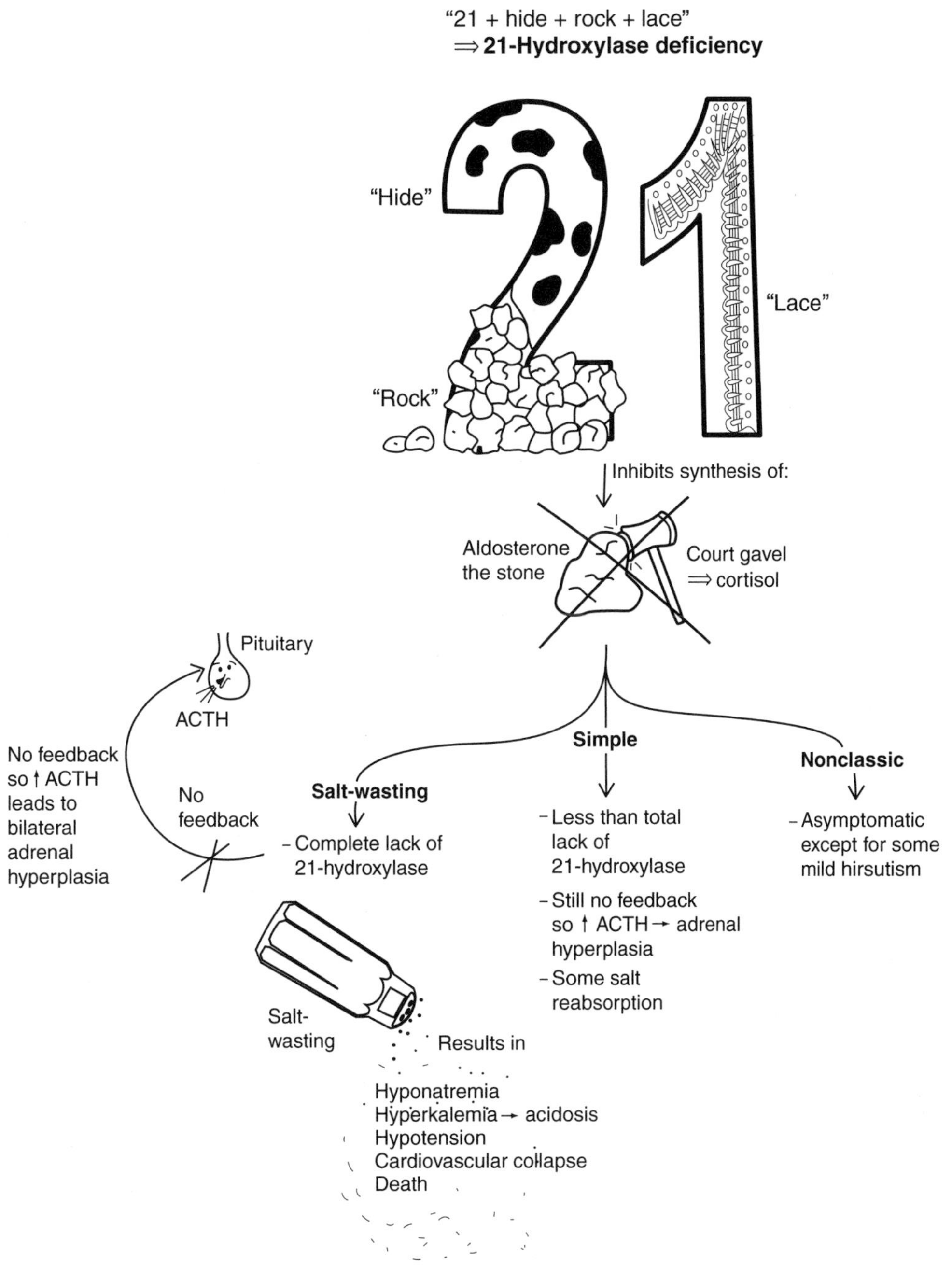

"21 + hide + rock + lace"
⇒ **21-Hydroxylase deficiency**

"Hide"

"Lace"

"Rock"

Inhibits synthesis of:

Aldosterone
the stone

Court gavel
⇒ cortisol

Pituitary

ACTH

No feedback
so ↑ ACTH
leads to
bilateral
adrenal
hyperplasia

No
feedback

Salt-wasting
↓
- Complete lack of
21-hydroxylase

Simple
↓
- Less than total
lack of
21-hydroxylase
- Still no feedback
so ↑ ACTH → adrenal
hyperplasia
- Some salt
reabsorption

Nonclassic
↓
- Asymptomatic
except for some
mild hirsutism

Salt-
wasting

Results in

Hyponatremia
Hyperkalemia → acidosis
Hypotension
Cardiovascular collapse
Death

NOTES

ADRENAL INSUFFICIENCY

- types: primary acute adrenocortical insufficiency (adrenal crisis); primary chronic adrenocortical insufficiency (Addison's disease); secondary adrenocortical insufficiency
- primary acute adrenocortical insufficiency: adrenal crisis occurs when a patient who already has chronic adrenocortical insufficiency cannot adequately react to stress because the adrenal glands are incapable of responding with immediate steroid output; when patients who take exogenous corticosteroids either rapidly withdraw from steroid use or do not increase steroid dose in response to acute stress; when there is massive adrenal hemorrhage (e.g., newborns following traumatic birth); patients on anticoagulant therapy; patients who have disseminated intravascular coagulation with resultant infarction of adrenals; and when massive adrenal hemorrhage complicates bacteremic infection (Waterhouse-Friderichsen syndrome)
- Waterhouse-Friderichsen syndrome: associated with overwhelming bacterial infection, usually *Neisseria meningitidis* septicemia; rapidly progressive hypotension leading to shock; disseminated intravascular coagulation with extensive purpura, especially of skin

Primary Chronic Adrenocortical Insufficiency (Addison's Disease)

- results from progressive destruction of the adrenal cortex; more common in white women
- 90% associated with autoimmune adrenalitis, tuberculosis, or metastatic cancers
- clinical: Addison's disease is not symptomatic until 90% of cortex is destroyed or nonfunctional; initially→ weakness and fatigue; gastrointestinal disturbances (anorexia, nausea, vomiting, weight loss, and diarrhea); hyperpigmentation of skin (from ACTH precursor hormones that stimulate melanocytes)

Secondary Adrenocortical Insufficiency

- disorder of hypothalamus and pituitary that reduces ACTH output or prolonged administration of exogenous glucocorticoids, which suppress ACTH release
- no hyperpigmentation
- characterized by deficient cortisol and androgen output but normal aldosterone synthesis (aldosterone being influenced by the renin system)

Adrenocortical Neoplasms

- most adenomas are nonfunctional
- carcinomas: occur at any age; functional; associated with symptoms of hyperadrenalism; highly malignant; strong propensity to invade adrenal vein, vena cava, and lymphatics

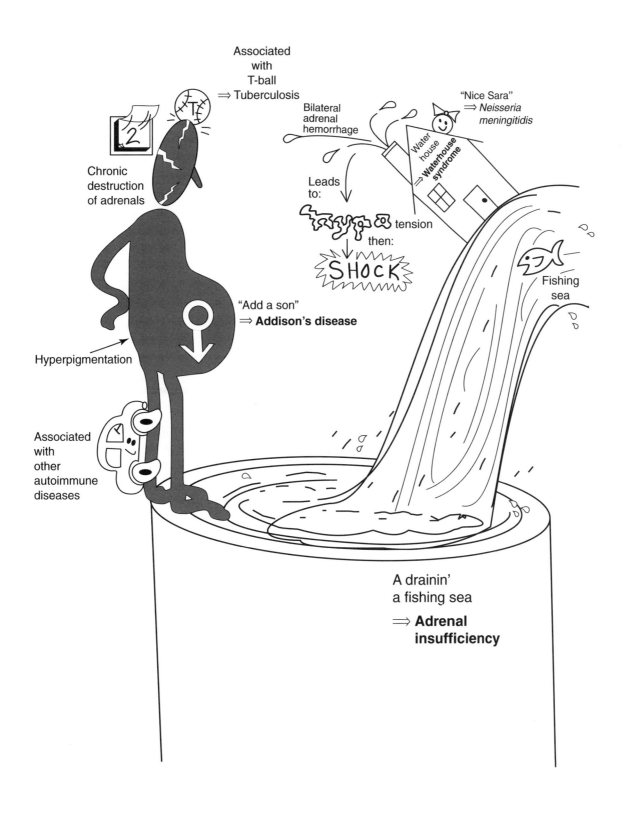

Associated
with
T-ball
⇒ Tuberculosis

Chronic
destruction
of adrenals

Hyperpigmentation

Associated
with
other
autoimmune
diseases

"Add a son"
⇒ **Addison's disease**

Bilateral
adrenal
hemorrhage

Leads
to:

tension

then:

SHOCK

"Nice Sara"
⇒ *Neisseria
meningitidis*

Water
house
**Waterhouse
syndrome**

Fishing
sea

A drainin'
a fishing sea

⇒ **Adrenal
insufficiency**

NOTES

ADRENAL MEDULLA

- composed of specialized neural crest (neuroendocrine) cells→chromaffin cells
- synthesize and secrete catecholamines (epinephrine and norepinephrine) in response to preganglionic sympathetic nervous system
- neuroendocrine cells can also produce other substances, such as histamine, serotonin, renin, chromogranin A, and neuropeptide hormones
- paraganglion system: neuroendocrine cells dispersed in an extra-adrenal system of clusters and nodules; closely associated with autonomic nervous system; divided according to anatomic position→branchiomeric, intravagal, aorticosympathetic; examples include carotid bodies

Pheochromocytoma

- neoplasms composed of chromaffin cells
- synthesize and release catecholamines and sometimes peptide hormones
- most arise in adrenal medulla but can also arise in extra-adrenal paraganglia, known as *paragangliomas* (more often below diaphragm)
- occurs sporadically or as familial syndrome (autosomal dominant and includes MEN syndromes, type I neurofibromatosis, von Hippel–Lindau disease, and Sturge-Weber syndrome)
- histology: composed of polygonal to spindle-shaped chromaffin cells, clustered with their supporting cells into small nests or alveoli (zellballen)
- diagnosis: based exclusively on the presence of metastases
- clinical: dominant symptom is hypertension, which is abrupt and associated with tachycardia, palpitations, headache, sweating, tremor, and sense of apprehension; catecholamine cardiomyopathy (catecholamine-induced myocardial instability and ventricular arrhythmias)
- laboratory diagnosis: increased urinary excretion of free catecholamines and their metabolites (vanillylmandelic acid [VMA] and metanephrines)

Neuroblastoma

- most common extracranial solid tumor of childhood; originates in adrenal medulla or anywhere in sympathetic nervous system; sporadic or familial

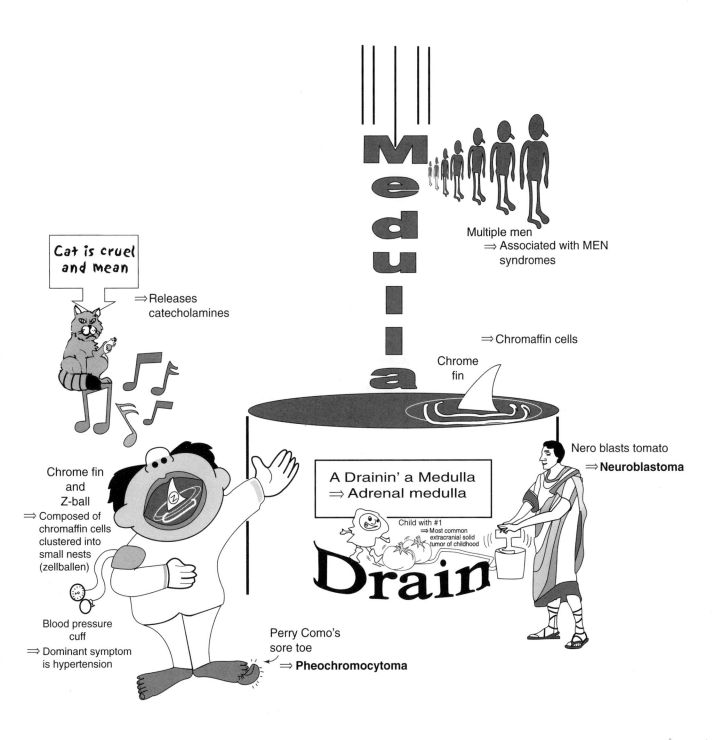

Cat is cruel and mean
⇒ Releases catecholamines

M e d u l l a

Multiple men
⇒ Associated with MEN syndromes

⇒ Chromaffin cells

Chrome fin

Chrome fin and Z-ball
⇒ Composed of chromaffin cells clustered into small nests (zellballen)

Blood pressure cuff
⇒ Dominant symptom is hypertension

A Drainin' a Medulla
⇒ Adrenal medulla

Drain

Child with #1
⇒ Most common extracranial solid tumor of childhood

Nero blasts tomato
⇒ **Neuroblastoma**

Perry Como's sore toe
⇒ **Pheochromocytoma**

NOTES

PINEAL GLAND ("PIN AN EEL")

- tumors are rare; most arise from sequestered embryonic germ cells (germinomas)
- pinealomas: two categories→ pineoblastomas and pineocytomas
- pineoblastomas→occur in young and invade surrounding tissue; rosettes present; tendency to spread via cerebrospinal fluid; mass may compress aqueduct of Sylvius and cause internal hydrocephalus; survival less than 2 years
- pineocytomas→slower growing; do not infiltrate; exhibit divergent glial and neuronal differentiation; pseudorosettes rimmed by rows of pineocytes are found

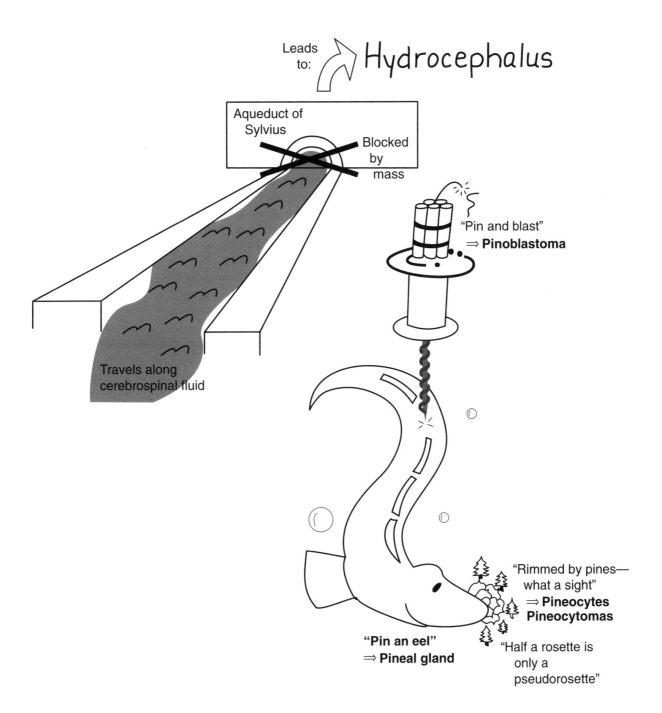

Leads to: Hydrocephalus

Aqueduct of Sylvius

Blocked by mass

Travels along cerebrospinal fluid

"Pin and blast"
⇒ **Pinoblastoma**

"Rimmed by pines—
what a sight"
⇒ **Pineocytes**
Pineocytomas

"Pin an eel"
⇒ **Pineal gland**

"Half a rosette is
only a
pseudorosette"

NOTES

⇒ Hyaline thickening of efferent and afferent arterioles, which is diagnostic for diabetes mellitus nephropathy

Clinical symptoms:

Hyaline hyena on road into glomerulus

Hyaline hyena on road out of glomerulus

Retinopathy and blindness

Dipstick
⇒ Proteinuria on dipstick UA

Also hematuria (color urine red)

Protein (steak) in urine

Glomerulus

⇒ #1 Systemic disease causing nephropathy

1

DIAGNOSTIC

Basement membrane thickening

BM

Linear deposition of IgG along glomerular walls
IgG IgG IgG IgG

GFR

Stages:

Causes microalbuminuria

"Microaluminum"

RIP

Increased BUN and protein

"Diet of beets"
⇒ **Diabetes mellitus**

End-stage renal disease

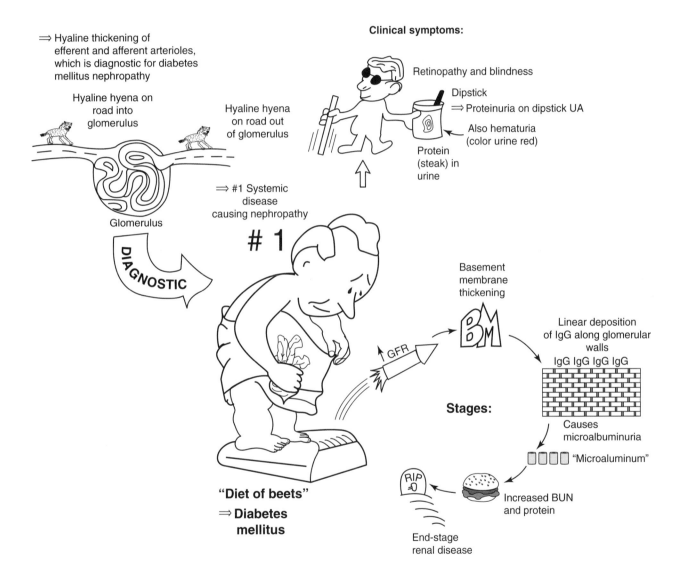

Differences Between Type I and Type II Diabetes Mellitis

NOTES

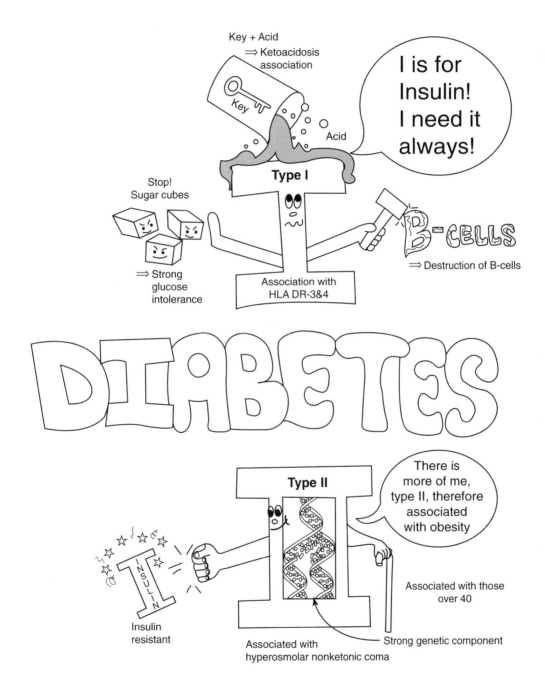

8.
BRAIN

INTRACRANIAL HEMORRHAGE

■ INTRACRANIAL HEMORRHAGE

- associated with hypertension

■ SUBARACHNOID HEMORRHAGE

⇒ spider
- most often involves rupture of a berry aneurysm
- patients report the "worst headache of their life"
  ⇒ berry holding head

Berry Aneurysm

- associated with adult polycystic kidney disease, Marfan's syndrome, and Ehlers-Danlos syndrome
  ⇒ kidneys on berry
- rupture may lead to subarachnoid hemorrhage, papilledema, and CN III palsy
  ⇒ CN III palsy⇒eye is down and out; CN III palsy⇒ptosis
- occurs at bifurcations in the circle of Willis
  ⇒ berry kicking Willis in a circle

Epidural Hematoma

- bleeding from middle meningeal artery
  ⇒ men in middle
- associated with fracture of temporal bone
- characterized clinically by a lucid interval
  lucid⇒moon

Subdural Hematoma

  ⇒ submarine
- bleeding from bridging veins
  ⇒ bridge
- characterized clinically by a gradual onset of symptoms

■ INFARCTION

- thrombosis caused by atherosclerosis
- embolism caused by valvular vegetations, air bubble, tumor cells, or fat
  - middle cerebral artery is the most common site of occlusion

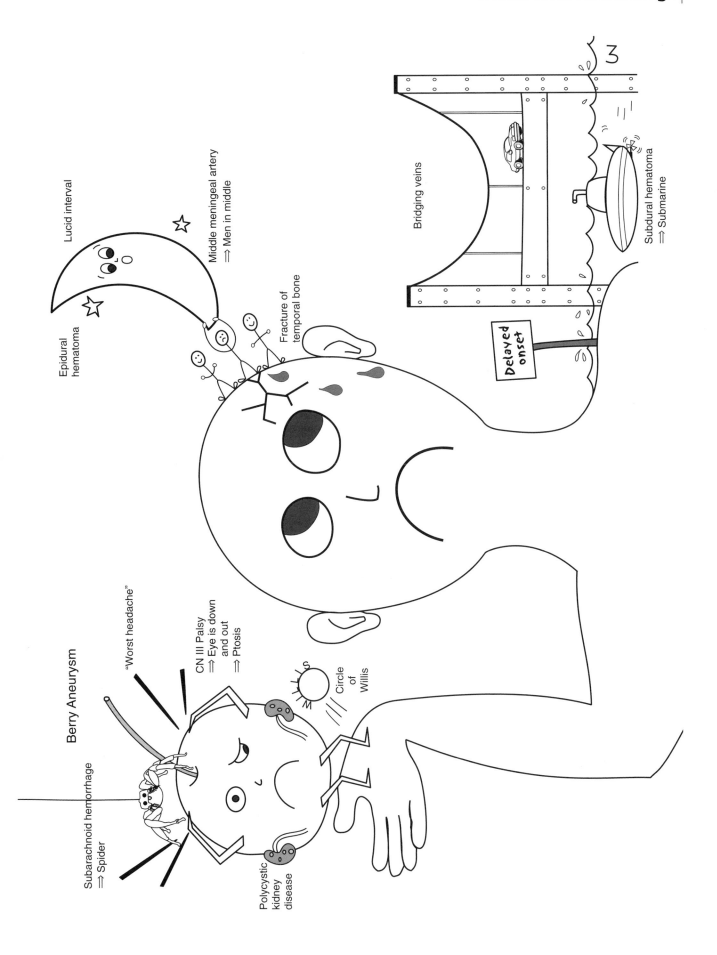

NOTES

ALZHEIMER'S DISEASE

- degenerative disease of the cerebral cortex
  cortex⇒apple core
- most common cause of dementia in the elderly
  dementia⇒Who? What? When?
- senile plaques contain β-amyloid core
  ⇒ Amy and Lloyd in plaque
- neurofibrillary tangles contain abnormal tau protein
  ⇒ tangled towel with steak (protein)
- Hirano bodies are eosinophilic inclusions of actin
  Hirano⇒he ran
- associated with alterations in nucleus basalis of Meynet
- decrease in acetylcholine in cerebral cortex and hippocampus
  ⇒ ACh falling down
- increased incidence in Down syndrome patients
- associated with chromosomes 1, 14, 19, and 21
  chromosomes⇒crow
- apolipoprotein E4 allele
- earliest symptom includes loss of recent memory
  ⇒ Who? What? When?

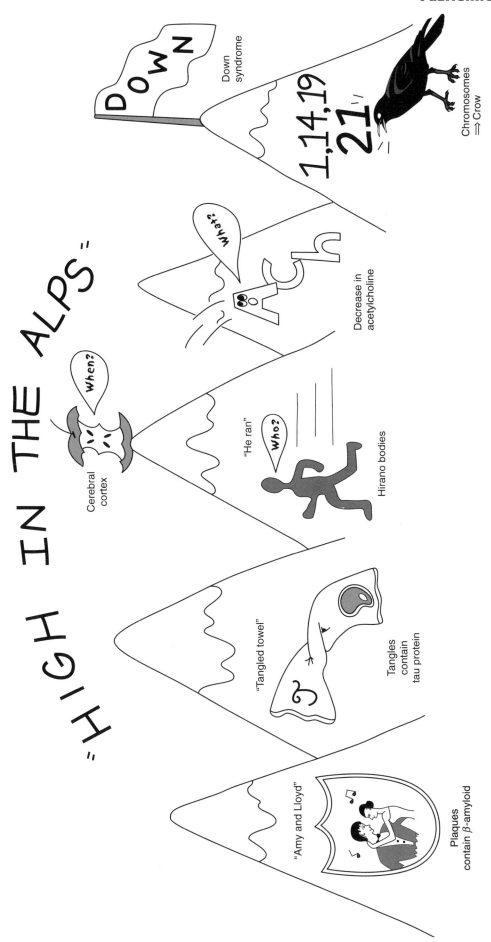

NOTES

PARKINSON'S DISEASE

- ⇒ park
- onset usually after age 50
- associated with depigmentation of the substantia nigra
  substantia nigra⇒Niagara Falls
- degeneration of dopaminergic neurons in substantia
  - ⇒ dope
- resting pill-rolling tremor
- muscular rigidity
- expressionless facies
- shuffling gait
- stooped posture
- slow voluntary movements
- Lewy bodies present
  - ⇒ lure
- treatment with levodopa (L-dopa), a dopamine precursor⇒dope
- other causes include
  - trauma (seen in boxers)
    - ⇒ boxing glove
  - postencephalitic parkinsonism: seen in patients after influenza epidemic (1914–1918) concurrently infected with encephalitis
    influenza⇒in flew Enza the witch
  - drugs (MPTP in illicit drugs)

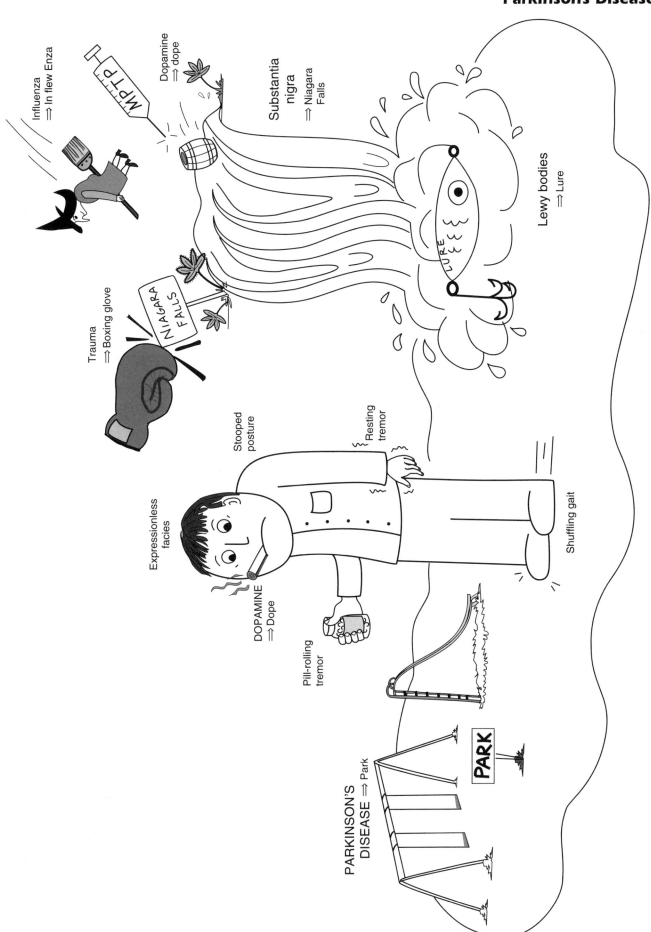

NOTES

OTHER DEGENERATIVE CENTRAL NERVOUS SYSTEM (CNS) DISEASES

Pick's Disease

- atrophy of the frontal and temporal lobes
  - ⇒ pick striking front of head
- pick bodies are present and consist of neurofilaments
- more common in women

Huntington's Disease

  - ⇒ hunter
- atrophy of caudate nucleus
  - ⇒ caudate⇒codfish
- autosomal dominant disorder
- defect on chromosome 4
- onset at 30–40 years of age; fatal
- choreiform movements
  - ⇒ dancin'
- dementia and incontinence
- affects gamma-aminobutyric acid (GABA) and cholinergic acetylcholine (ACh) neurons

Friedrich's Ataxia

  - ⇒ Fried Rich's taxi
- degeneration of posterior columns and corticospinal tract
- autosomal recessive, more males than females
- adolescent onset, death in 30s
- progressive ataxia
  - ⇒ taxi
- associated with myocarditis and diabetes
  diabetes⇒diet of beets

Amyotrophic Lateral Sclerosis (ALS)

- also known as *Lou Gehrig's disease*
  - ⇒ baseball player
- upper and lower motor neurons affected
  - ⇒ upper and lower baseballs
- degeneration of anterior motor neurons and lateral corticospinal tracts
  anterior motor neurons⇒ant
- onset in middle age; rapid course; fatal in 1 to 5 years
- lower motor neuron signs include weakness and atrophy of musculature
- upper motor neuron signs include hyperreflexia

Werdnig-Hoffman Disease

  - ⇒ "We're diggin' off"
- floppy baby syndrome
- autosomal recessive
- lower motor neurons affected
- death within months from respiratory failure

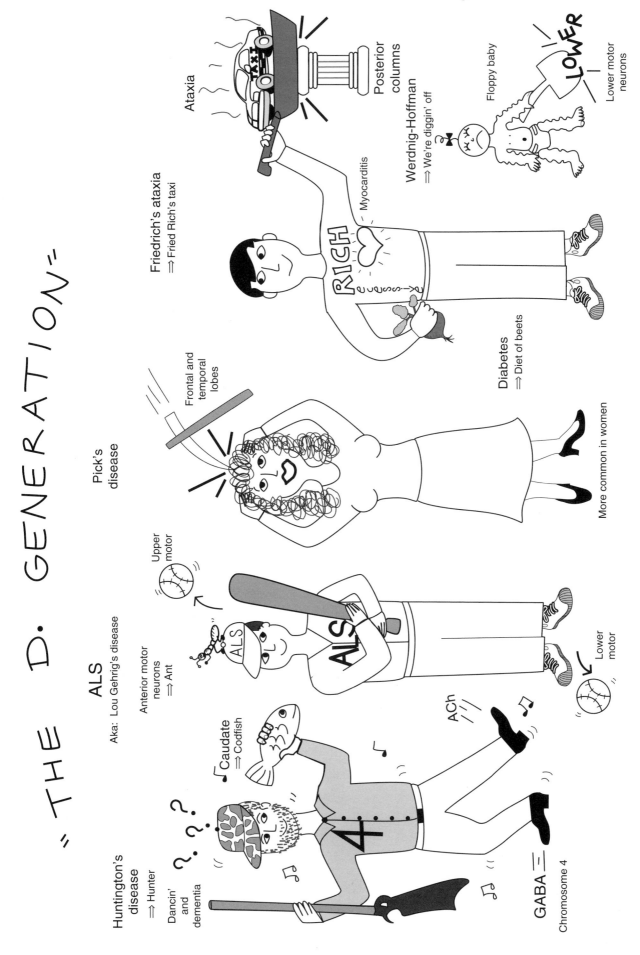

"THE D. GENERATION"

Ataxia

Posterior columns

Friedrich's ataxia
⇒ Fried Rich's taxi

Myocarditis

Werdnig-Hoffman
⇒ We're diggin' off

Floppy baby

Lower motor neurons

RICH

Diabetes
⇒ Diet of beets

Pick's disease

Frontal and temporal lobes

More common in women

ALS
Aka: Lou Gehrig's disease

Anterior motor neurons
⇒ Ant

Upper motor

ALS

Lower motor

Huntington's disease
⇒ Hunter

Dancin' and dementia

Caudate
⇒ Codfish

ACh

GABA

Chromosome 4

NOTES

DEMYELINATING DISEASES

- ⇒ myelin around axon damaged
- myelin production
  - peripheral nervous system (PNS): Schwann cells
  - CNS: oligodendrocytes

Multiple Sclerosis

- ⇒ multiple scares (ghosts)
- more common in women and whites in northern latitudes
  women⇒bows
- onset 20–40 years of age
- formation of plaques (demyelinated areas)
- affects periventricular areas, optic nerve, brain stem, and spinal cord
- sparing of axons, loss of oligodendrocytes
  - ⇒ igloo running away
- reactive gliosis occurs
  gliosis⇒glee (smiley face)
- increased immunoglobulin (Ig) in cerebrospinal fluid (CSF)
- unkown etiology; environmental and genetic factors
- relapsing and remitting course
- Charcot's triad of symptoms:
  - ⇒ charcoal triad
  - nystagmus
    - ⇒ eyes with arrows
  - scanning speech
    - ⇒ coal says "scan"
  - intention tremor
    - ⇒ coal with tremor
- other clinical manifestations include paresthesias, weakness, visual disturbances, and incontinence
  incontinence⇒ghost urinating
- often leads to paraplegia and mental dysfunction (⇒)

Guillain-Barré Syndrome (Acute Idiopathic Polyneuritis)

- ⇒ Gill the fish at the bar
- demyelination and inflammation of peripheral nerves
  - ⇒ "PERIPHERAL" around periphery of Gill the fish
- associated with preceding viral infections and immunizations
- CSF finding: albuminocytologic dissociation describes a normal cell count with elevated protein
  - ⇒ record album dissociating from cyto
- leads to symmetric ascending muscle weakness starting in distal lower extremities
  - ⇒ elevators going up in lower legs

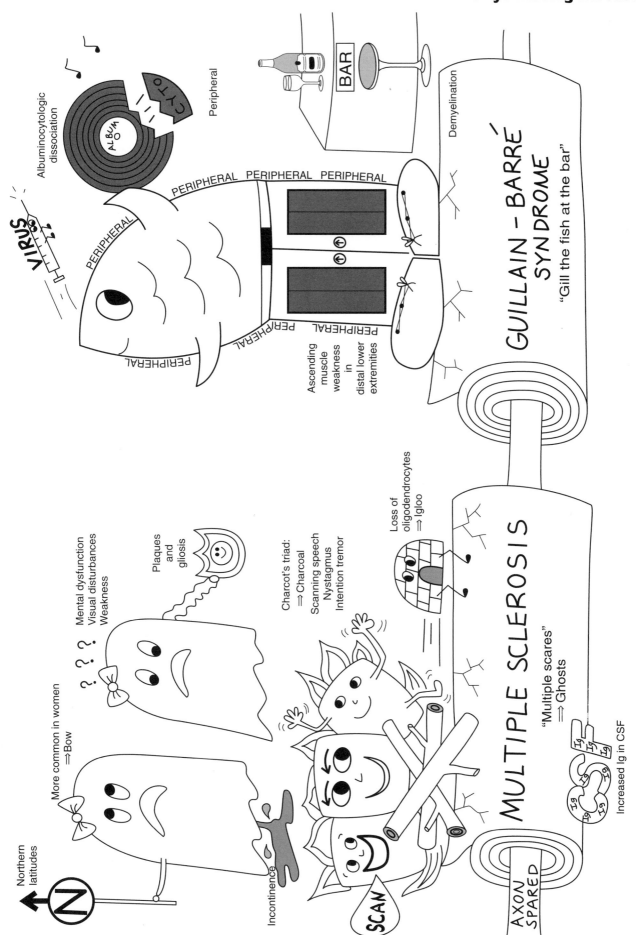

NOTES

WERNICKE-KORSAKOFF SYNDROME

⇒ icky worm—coarse cough
- alcohol-induced thiamine deficiency
  alcohol⇒drinking beer; thiamine deficiency⇒"Where's my thigh?"
- Wernicke's triad: mental confusion, nystagmus, and ataxia
  confustion⇒???; nystagmus⇒eyes with arrows; ataxia⇒taxi
- Wernicke's involves lesions in the mammillary bodies
  mammillary⇒breast
- Wernicke's encephalopathy may progress to Korsakoff's psychosis without thiamine treatment
- Korsakoff's psychosis involves amnesia and lesions in the dorsal medial thalamic nuclei
  thalamic⇒"the Lamb"

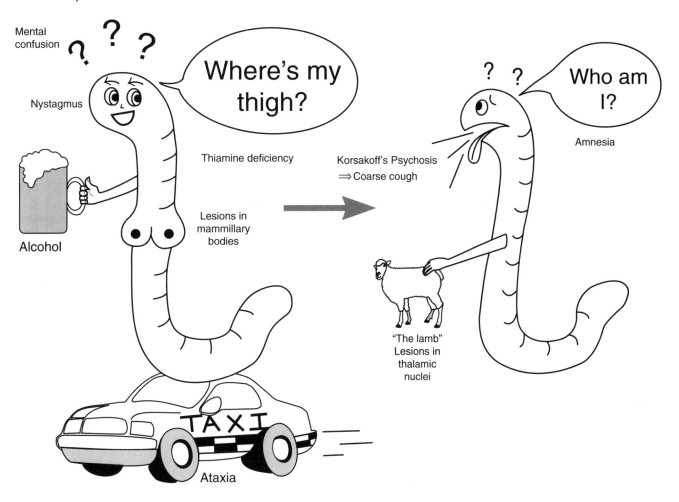

NOTES

SLOW VIRUS INFECTIONS OF CNS

Creutzfeldt-Jakob Disease

- ⇒ crew in the field
- possibly caused by prions
- spongiform encephalopathy present
  - ⇒ sponge
- leads to progressive dementia and death
- transmitted by tissue products
  - ⇒ facial tissue

Progressive Multifocal Leukoencephalopathy (PML)

- ⇒ locomotive with multifocal glasses
- caused by JC virus, a papovirus
  JC⇒junior chirper
- oligodendrocytes affected
  - ⇒ igloo
- causes focal demyelinating lesions
  - ⇒ myelin coming off axon
- often seen in patients with immunodeficiency, leukemia, or lymphoma

Kuru

- transmitted by ingestion
- seen in New Guinea
- spongiform encephalopathy present
- death within months

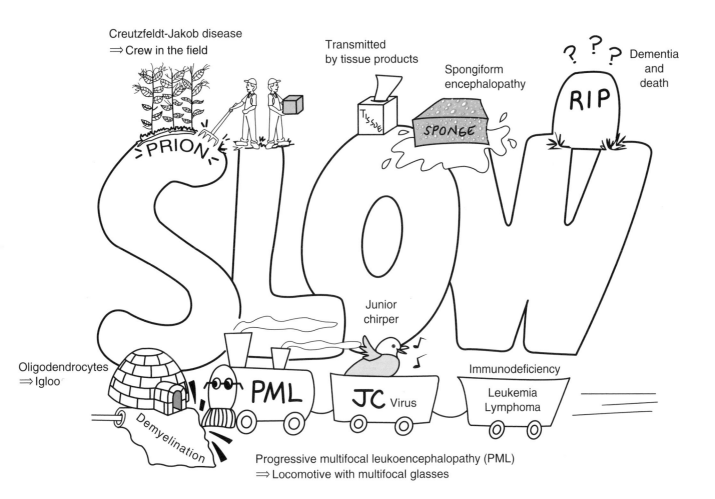

Creutzfeldt-Jakob disease ⇒ Crew in the field

Transmitted by tissue products

Spongiform encephalopathy

Dementia and death

Oligodendrocytes ⇒ Igloo

Junior chirper

Immunodeficiency

Leukemia Lymphoma

Progressive multifocal leukoencephalopathy (PML) ⇒ Locomotive with multifocal glasses

NOTES

GENETIC DISORDERS OF CNS (AUTOSOMAL DOMINANT)

Neurofibromatosis (von Recklinghausen's Disease)

⇒ van wrecking house
- characterized by neurofibromas, acoustic schwannomas, and meningiomas
  acoustic schwannomas⇒swan with ear
- multiple café au lait spots present
  ⇒ cup of coffee
- lisch nodules, which are pigmented hamartomas of the iris, are characteristic
  Lisch⇒list
- skeletal disorders may be present
- increased occurrence of other tumors including pheochromocytoma and rhabdomyosarcomas

Tuberous Sclerosis

⇒ tuba scare
- triad: angiofibromas, seizures, mental retardation
- cutaneous lesions include angiofibromas, shagreen patches, and ash-leaf patches
  ⇒ leaf and patch on ghost
- other findings include renal angiomyolipomas, retinal hamartomas, cardiac rhabdomyomas

von Hippel–Lindau Disease

⇒ van and hippo
- characterized by hemangioblastomas of the retina, brain stem, or cerebellum and visceral cysts
  ⇒ he-man blasting; retina⇒eye; cerebellum⇒bell
- increased risk of renal cell carcinoma
  ⇒ kidney on can of CANCER

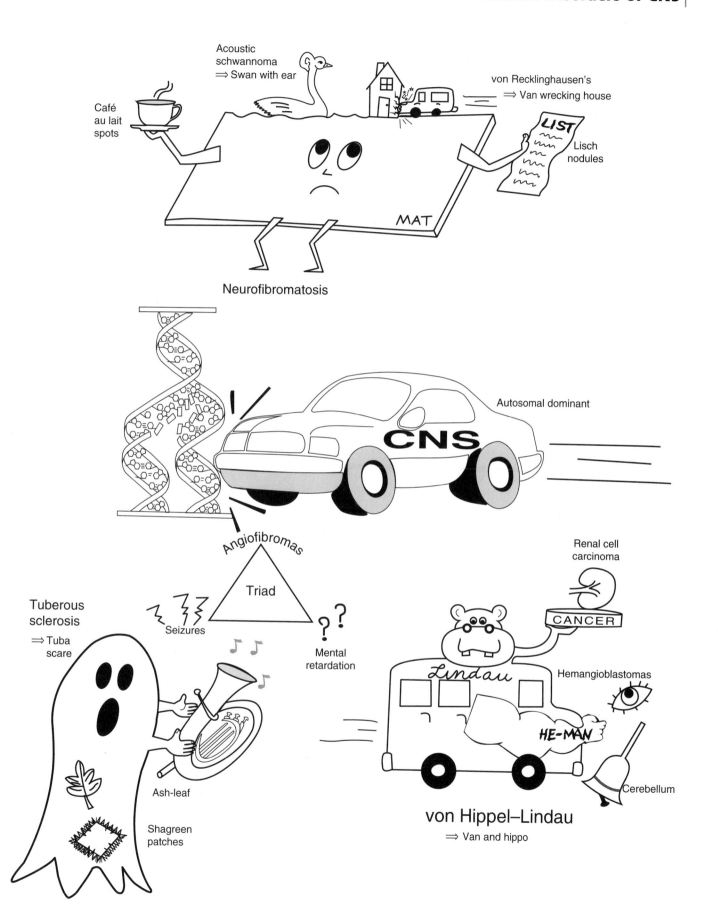

Café au lait spots

Acoustic schwannoma ⇒ Swan with ear

von Recklinghausen's ⇒ Van wrecking house

LIST

Lisch nodules

MAT

Neurofibromatosis

Autosomal dominant

CNS

Angiofibromas

Triad

Seizures

Mental retardation

Tuberous sclerosis ⇒ Tuba scare

Ash-leaf

Shagreen patches

Renal cell carcinoma

CANCER

Lindau

Hemangioblastomas

HE-MAN

Cerebellum

von Hippel–Lindau ⇒ Van and hippo

NOTES

- supratentorial
  - ⇒ above the tent

Glioblastoma Multiforme (Grade IV Astrocytoma)

Glioblastoma multiforme⇒glee = smiley face, boom = blast
Grade IV astrocytoma⇒astro star
- most common primary brain tumor
- occurs in cerebral hemispheres
- "pseudopalisading" tumor cells surround areas of necrosis and hemorrhage
- poor prognosis with death within 1 year

Meningioma

- ⇒ men in G
- second most common primary brain tumor
- benign tumor occurring more frequently in women
  women⇒bows
- arises from arachnoid cells
  arachnoid⇒spider
- found external to brain convexities of cerebral hemispheres parasagittal areas
- characterized by psammoma bodies (whorled pattern of spindle cells)
  psammoma⇒salmon

Schwannoma (Neurilemmoma)

- ⇒ swan
- third most common primary brain tumor
- benign encapsulated tumor of Schwann cell origin
  encapsulated⇒cap
- frequently localized to eighth cranial nerve (CN) and known as *acoustic neuroma*
  acoustic neuroma⇒ear
- characterized by Antoni A (compact cell pattern with palisading nuclei) and Antoni B (looser pattern)
  Antoni A B⇒ant on A B

Oligodendroglioma

- ⇒ igloo
- slow-growing, benign brain tumor
- characterized by sheets of cells with round nuclei and a clear halo of cytoplasm—"fried egg" appearance
- capillary network, calcifications found

Metastatic Brain Tumors

- half of intracranial tumors
- primary sites include lung, breast, skin, kidney, gastrointestinal, and thyroid

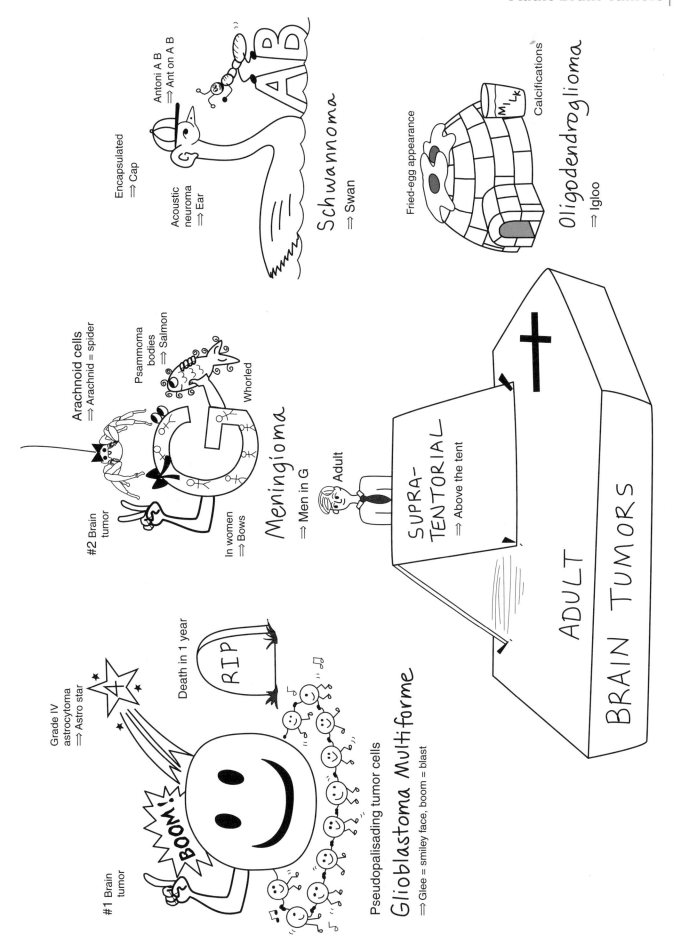

Schwannoma
⇒ Swan

Encapsulated
⇒ Cap

Acoustic
neuroma ⇒ Ear

Antoni A B
⇒ Ant on A B

Oligodendroglioma
⇒ Igloo

Fried-egg appearance

Calcifications

MILK

Meningioma
⇒ Men in G

Arachnoid cells
⇒ Arachnid = spider

Psammoma
bodies
⇒ Salmon

Whorled

#2 Brain
tumor

In women
⇒ Bows

Adult

SUPRA-
TENTORIAL
⇒ Above the tent

ADULT
BRAIN TUMORS

Glioblastoma Multiforme
⇒ Glee = smiley face, boom = blast

Grade IV
astrocytoma
⇒ Astro star

Death in 1 year

RIP

Pseudopalisading tumor cells

#1 Brain
tumor

BOOM!

CHILDHOOD BRAIN TUMORS

- ⇒ child on tomb
- infra-tentorial
  - ⇒ child in the tent

Medulloblastoma

- ⇒ blast with medal
- highly malignant tumor of the cerebellum
  cerebellum⇒bell
- characterized by sheets of cells in a rosette pattern
  - ⇒ roses
- a type of primitive neuroectodermal tumor (PNET)
  - ⇒ a P net
- may compress fourth ventricle leading to hydrocephalus
  hydrocephalus⇒hydrant

Meningioma

- ⇒ pen
- occurs most commonly in the fourth ventricle leading to hydrocephalus
  hydrocephalus⇒hydrant
- characterized by perivascular rosettes and rod-shaped blepharoblasts (basal bodies of cilia)
  - ⇒ roses, fishing rod

Hemangioblastoma

- ⇒ he-man blasting
- occurs most often in cerebellum
  - ⇒ bell
- associated with von Hippel–Lindau syndrome
  - ⇒ van with hippo
- characterized by foamy cells
  - ⇒ soap
- may produce erythropoietin leading to polycythemia
  erythropoietin⇒EPO

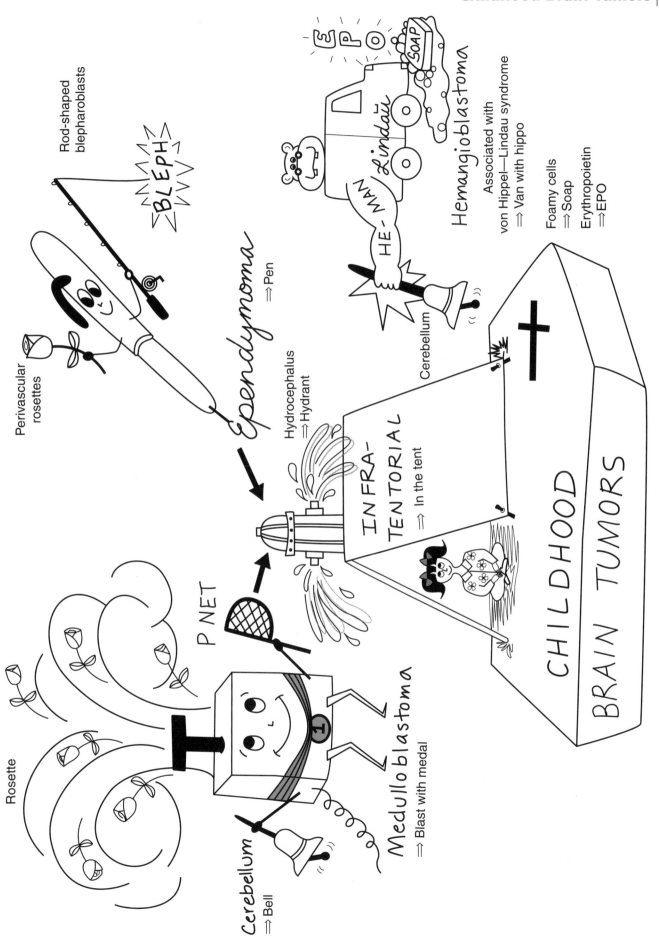

Rod-shaped blepharoblasts

≥BLEPH≥

Perivascular rosettes

Ependymoma
⇒ Pen

Hemangioblastoma
Associated with von Hippel—Lindau syndrome
⇒ Van with hippo

Foamy cells
⇒ Soap

Erythropoietin
⇒ EPO

HE—MAN

Lindau

SOAP

EPO

Cerebellum

Hydrocephalus
⇒ Hydrant

INFRA-TENTORIAL
⇒ In the tent

CHILDHOOD BRAIN TUMORS

PNET

Rosette

Medulloblastoma
⇒ Blast with medal

Cerebellum
⇒ Bell

9.
MALE GENITAL TRACT

NOTES

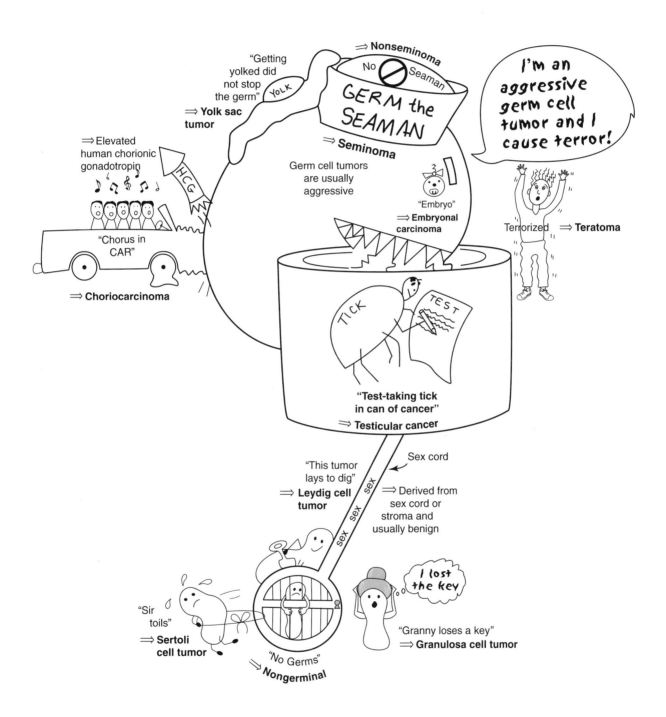

NOTES

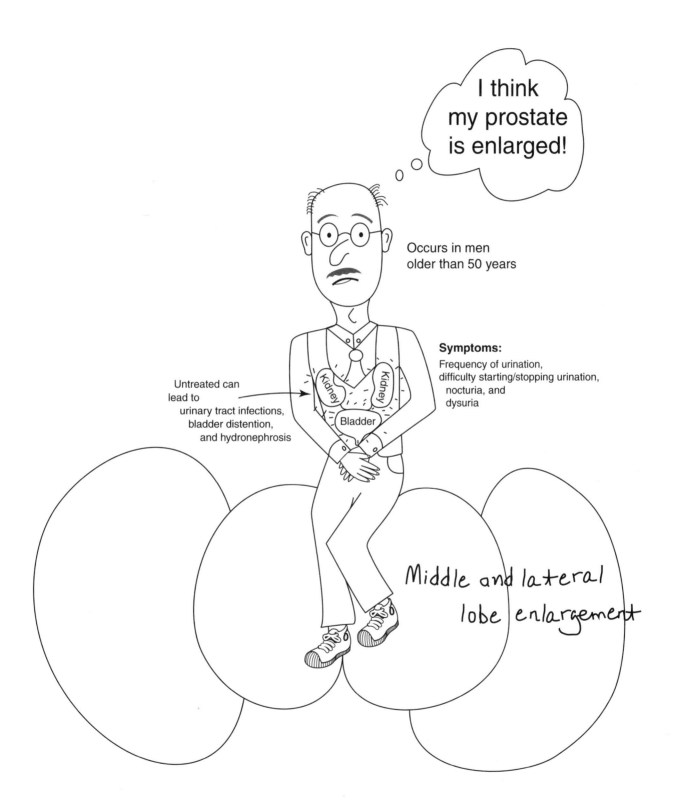

10.
FEMALE GENITAL TRACT

POLYCYSTIC OVARIAN SYNDROME (STEIN-LEVENTHAL)

- increased luteinizing hormone (LH) secretions lead to anovulation
  ⇒ left hand up
- found in young women
- thickened ovarian capsule present
  ⇒ egg in cap
- patients present with amenorrhea, hirsutism, infertility, and obesity
  amenorrhea⇒"no need for tampons"; hirsutism⇒beard; infertility⇒no baby on board
- treatment includes oral contraceptives (OCP), weight loss, or surgery

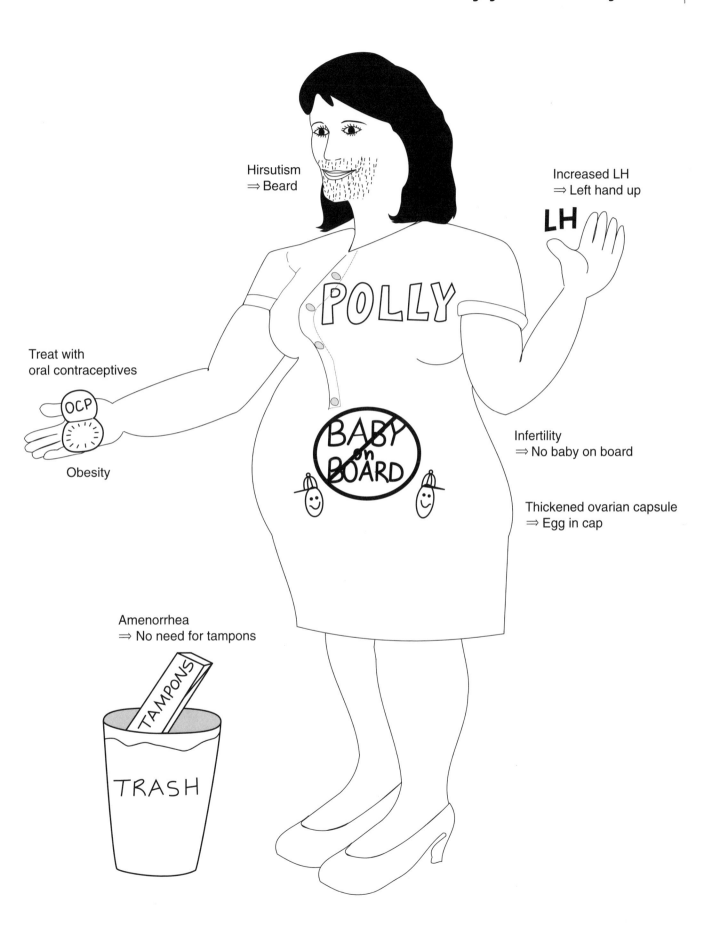

Hirsutism
⇒ Beard

Increased LH
⇒ Left hand up

LH

Treat with
oral contraceptives

OCP

Obesity

Infertility
⇒ No baby on board

Thickened ovarian capsule
⇒ Egg in cap

Amenorrhea
⇒ No need for tampons

TAMPONS

TRASH

POLLY

BABY on BOARD

NOTES

ENDOMETRIOSIS

- ⇒ in dome
- endometrial tissue outside of uterus (nonneoplastic)
- ovaries most common site of ectopic tissue
  - ⇒ basket of eggs
- patients present with dysmenorrhea, chronic pelvic pain, and infertility
- results in blood-filled "chocolate" cysts

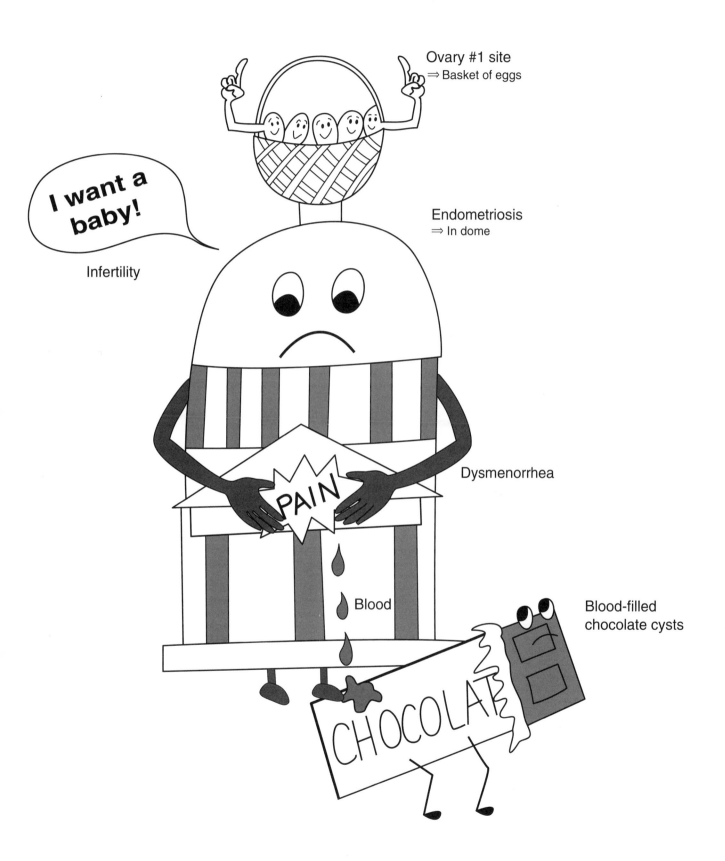

NOTES

⇒ Leo the lion

- benign tumor of myometrium
  benign⇒bee 9
- known as *fibroids*
- most common tumor in women
- increased incidence in black women
- estrogen sensitive: rapid growth during pregnancy and decreases with menopause
  estrogen sensitive⇒astro jeans
- patients present with vaginal bleeding and pain

Leiomyosarcoma

- malignant tumor of myometrium
- increased incidence in black women
- frequent recurrence
- does not arise from leiomyoma
- areas of necrosis and hemorrhage present

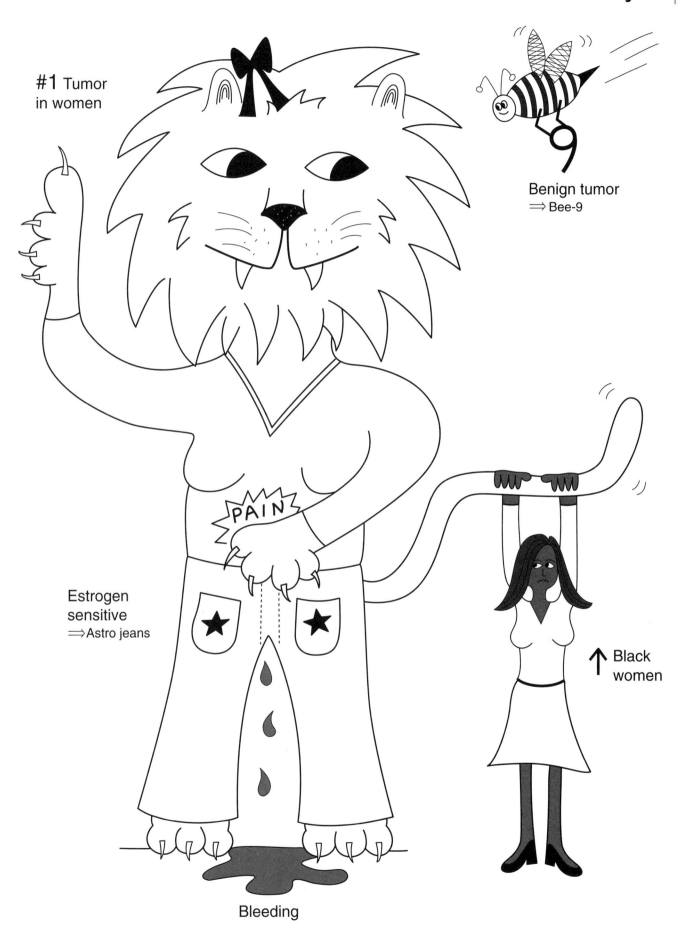

#1 Tumor
in women

Benign tumor
⟹ Bee-9

Estrogen
sensitive
⟹Astro jeans

PAIN

Black
women

Bleeding

NOTES

HYDATIDIFORM MOLE

- occurs in the early months of pregnancy
- cystic swelling of chorionic villi
  - ⇒ villain
- trophoblastic proliferation
  - ⇒ trophy
- high β-HCG (human chorionic gonadotropin)
- precursor of choriocarcinoma
  - ⇒ core
- resembles a cluster of grapes
- presents with uterine bleeding
- a complete mole is exclusively paternal and has no fetal remnants
  paternal⇒#1 Dad; no fetal remnants⇒no baby
- a partial mole is triploid or tetraploid, and fetal remnants are present
  partial mole⇒part of a mole; fetal remnants present⇒baby

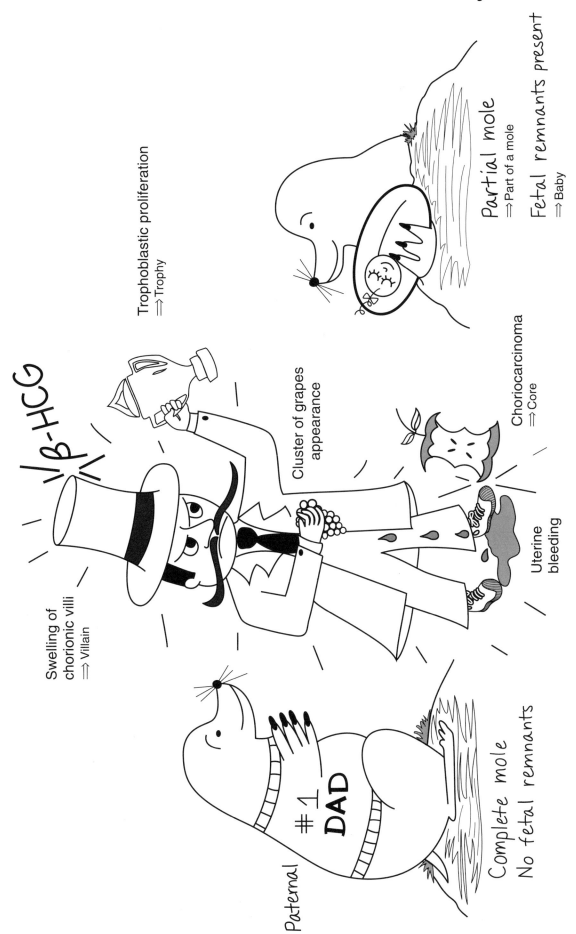

Trophoblastic proliferation
⇒ Trophy

Partial mole
⇒ Part a mole

Fetal remnants present
⇒ Baby

β-HCG

Cluster of grapes
appearance

Choriocarcinoma
⇒ Core

Swelling of
chorionic villi
⇒ Villain

Uterine
bleeding

Paternal

#1 DAD

Complete mole
No fetal remnants

NOTES

FIBROCYSTIC BREAST DISEASE

- most common type of palpable breast mass in patients between ages 25 and 50
  - ⇒ hand feeling bra
- often bilateral
- patients present with breast tenderness and multiple lumps
- usually does not indicate an increased risk of cancer
- increased risk of cancer when hyperplastic epithelium shows atypia
  - ⇒ hyper plastic shows type A on can of CANCER
- characterized by fluid-filled cysts (blue-dome cysts), fibrosis, and epithelial changes
  - ⇒ fluid-filled domes; fibrosis⇒fibers
- sclerosing adenosis (the increase in acini combined with fibrosis) may occur
  - ⇒ scary, add

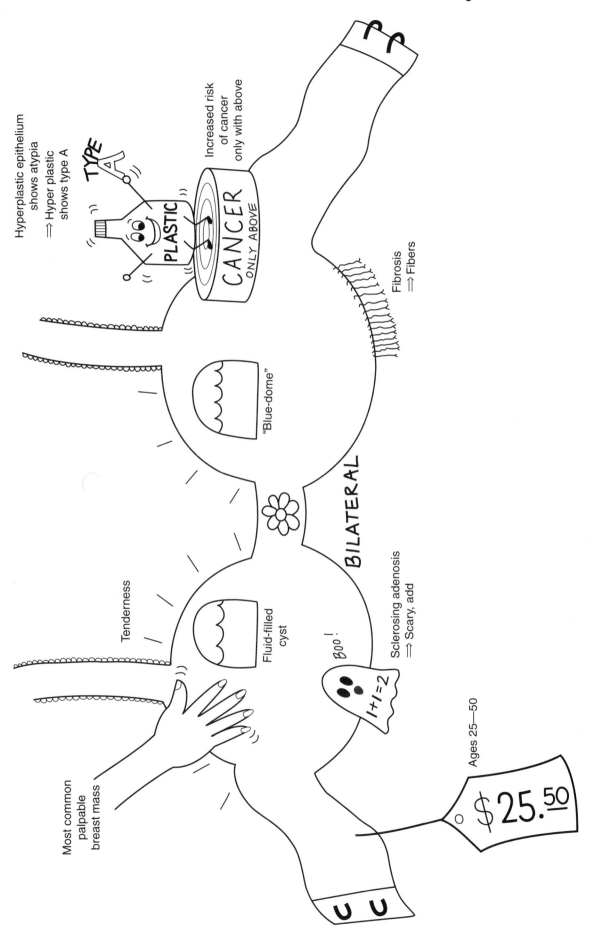

NOTES

BENIGN TUMORS OF THE BREAST

⇒ bee 9

- fibroadenoma
  - ⇒ add = plus sign, bro
  - most common breast tumor under age 25
  - small, firm, well-circumscribed, mobile mass
  - painless
  - ⇒ band-aid
- intraductal papilloma
  - ⇒ duck on pillow
  - lactiferous duct tumor
    - ⇒ milk
  - presents with serous or bloody nipple discharge
- phyllodes tumor
  - ⇒ Phyllis
  - large cystic mass of connective tissue
  - characterized by "leaflike" appearance of breast surface

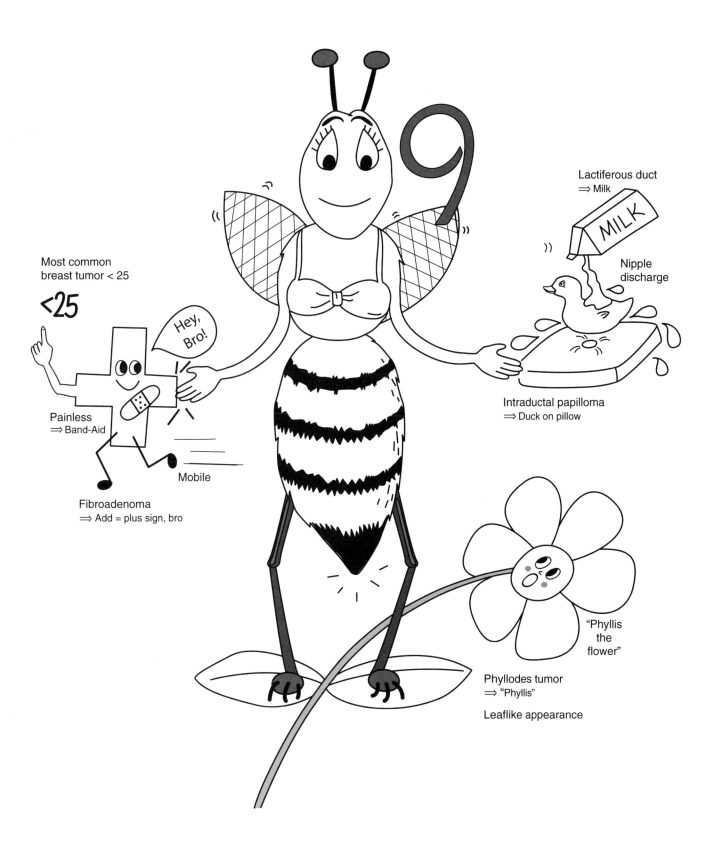

Most common breast tumor < 25

<25

Hey, Bro!

Painless
⇒ Band-Aid

Mobile

Fibroadenoma
⇒ Add = plus sign, bro

Lactiferous duct
⇒ Milk

Nipple discharge

Intraductal papilloma
⇒ Duck on pillow

"Phyllis the flower"

Phyllodes tumor
⇒ "Phyllis"

Leaflike appearance

NOTES

CARCINOMA OF THE BREAST

⇒ can of CANCER in bra
- second most common malignancy found in women (lung cancer number 1)
- most frequently found in the upper outer quadrant of the breast
  ⇒ hands are upper and outer
- estrogen and progesterone receptors may be present and indicate a better prognosis
  estrogen receptors⇒astro jeans
- comedocarcinoma: necrosis with cheeselike consistency
  ⇒ comedian
- Paget's disease of the breast: eczematous lesions on the nipple
  Paget's⇒pageant = crown; eczematous lesions of the nipple⇒Ax Emma
- inflammatory carcinoma: lymphatic involvement leading to pain, swelling, peau d'orange appearance to skin
  ⇒ orange in flames
- invasive ductal carcinoma: firm, fibrous, most common carcinoma of the breast
  ⇒ invading duck
- risk factors include age, early menarche, late menopause, late first pregnancy, nulliparity, family history of first-degree relative, cancer in one breast, and fibrocystic disease with atypical epithelial hyperplasia

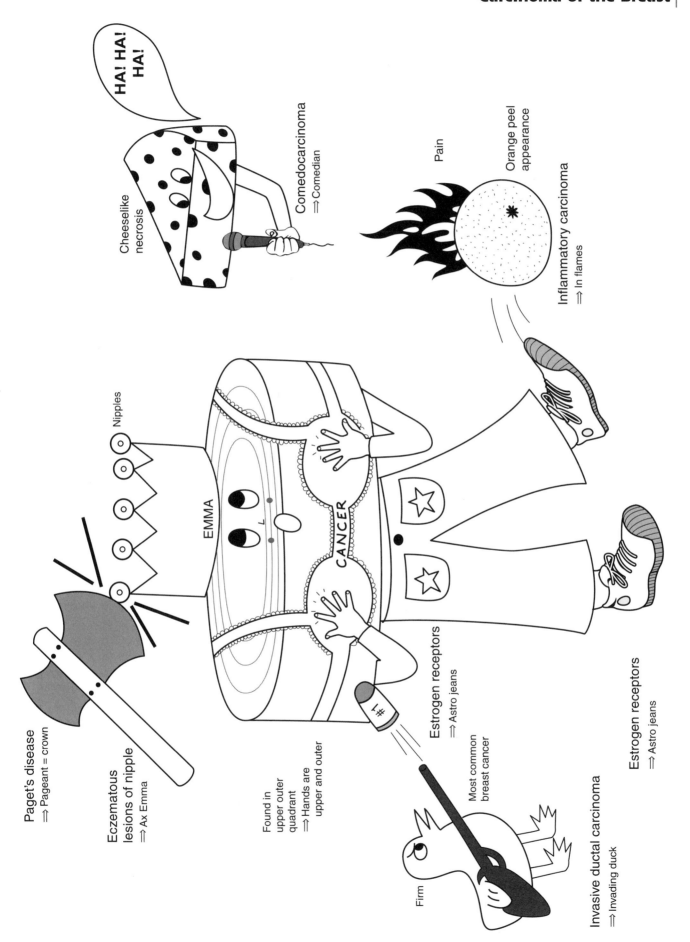

11.
SKELETAL SYSTEM

NOTES

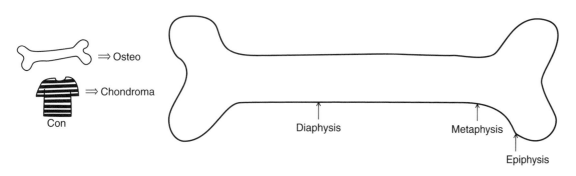

⇒ Osteo

⇒ Chondroma

Con

Diaphysis

Metaphysis

Epiphysis

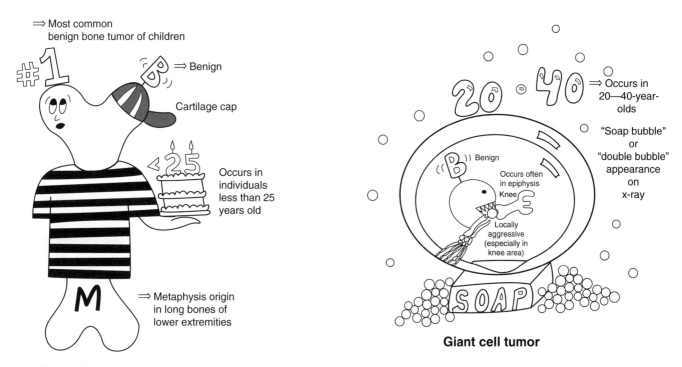

⇒ Most common
   benign bone tumor of children

⇒ Benign

Cartilage cap

< 25

Occurs in
individuals
less than 25
years old

M

⇒ Metaphysis origin
   in long bones of
   lower extremities

Osteochondroma

"Osteo con"

20   40 ⇒ Occurs in
             20—40-year-
             olds

Benign

Occurs often
in epiphysis
Knee

Locally
aggressive
(especially in
knee area)

"Soap bubble"
or
"double bubble"
appearance
on
x-ray

SOAP

Giant cell tumor

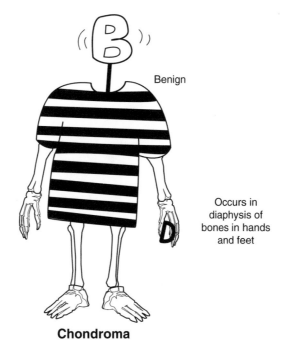

Benign

Occurs in
diaphysis of
bones in hands
and feet

D

Chondroma

NOTES

⇒ Osteo

⇒ Sarcoma

Arc

"Sock with arc"

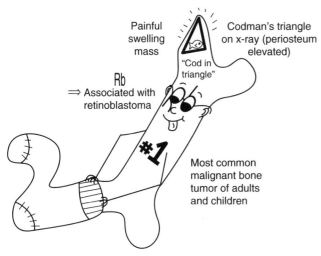

Painful swelling mass

Codman's triangle on x-ray (periosteum elevated)

"Cod in triangle"

Rb

⇒ Associated with retinoblastoma

#1

Most common malignant bone tumor of adults and children

"Osteo putting on sock with arc"

⇒ **Osteosarcoma**

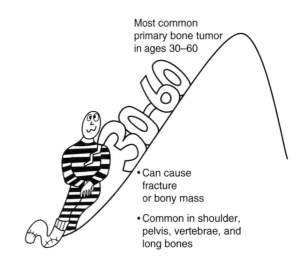

Most common primary bone tumor in ages 30–60

30-60

• Can cause fracture or bony mass

• Common in shoulder, pelvis, vertebrae, and long bones

"Con's sock with arc"

⇒ **Chondrosarcoma**

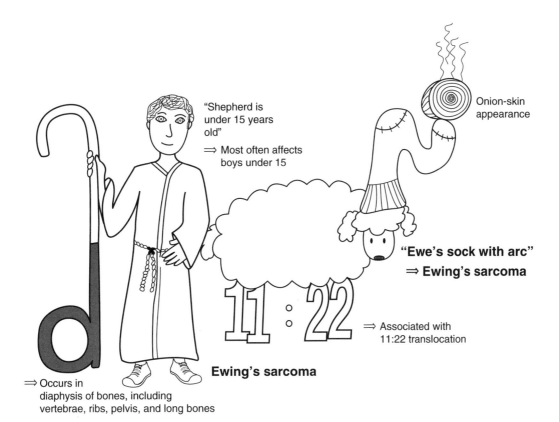

"Shepherd is under 15 years old"

⇒ Most often affects boys under 15

Onion-skin appearance

"Ewe's sock with arc"

⇒ **Ewing's sarcoma**

⇒ Associated with 11:22 translocation

Ewing's sarcoma

⇒ Occurs in diaphysis of bones, including vertebrae, ribs, pelvis, and long bones

NOTES

"OSTEO PORES"

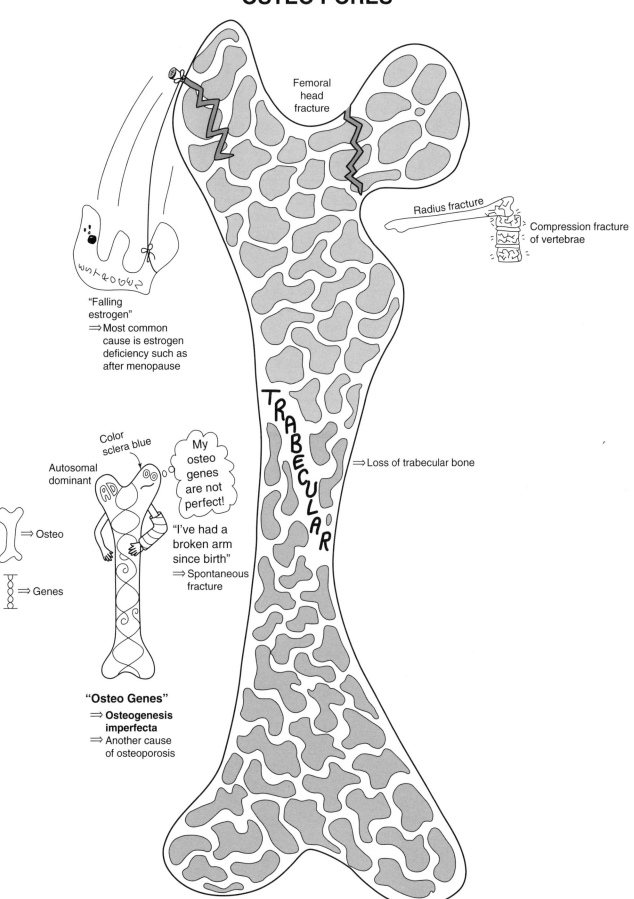

Femoral head fracture

Radius fracture

Compression fracture of vertebrae

"Falling estrogen"
⇒ Most common cause is estrogen deficiency such as after menopause

⇒ Loss of trabecular bone

TRABECULAR

Color sclera blue

Autosomal dominant

My osteo genes are not perfect!

"I've had a broken arm since birth"
⇒ Spontaneous fracture

⇒ Osteo

⇒ Genes

"Osteo Genes"
⇒ **Osteogenesis imperfecta**
⇒ Another cause of osteoporosis

NOTES

NOTES

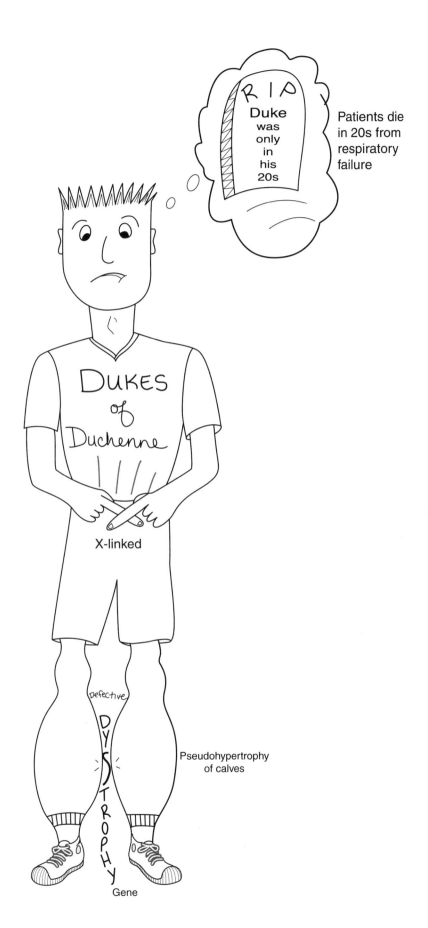

NOTES

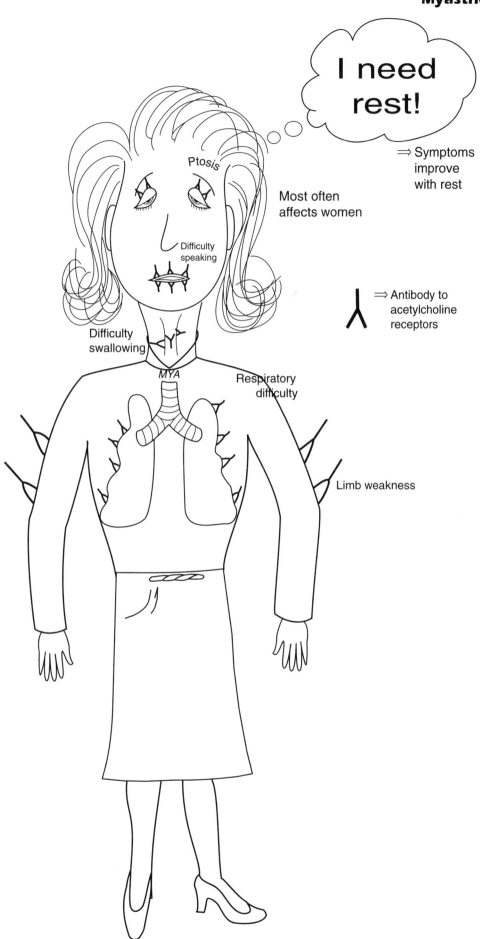

12.
DISEASE OF IMMUNITY

NOTES

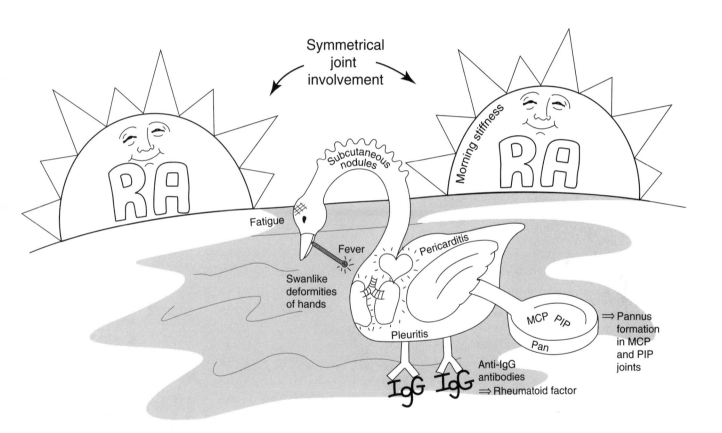

Symmetrical joint involvement

Morning stiffness

Subcutaneous nodules

Fatigue

Fever

Swanlike deformities of hands

Pericarditis

Pleuritis

Anti-IgG antibodies ⇒ Rheumatoid factor

IgG IgG

MCP PIP

Pan

⇒ Pannus formation in MCP and PIP joints

NOTES

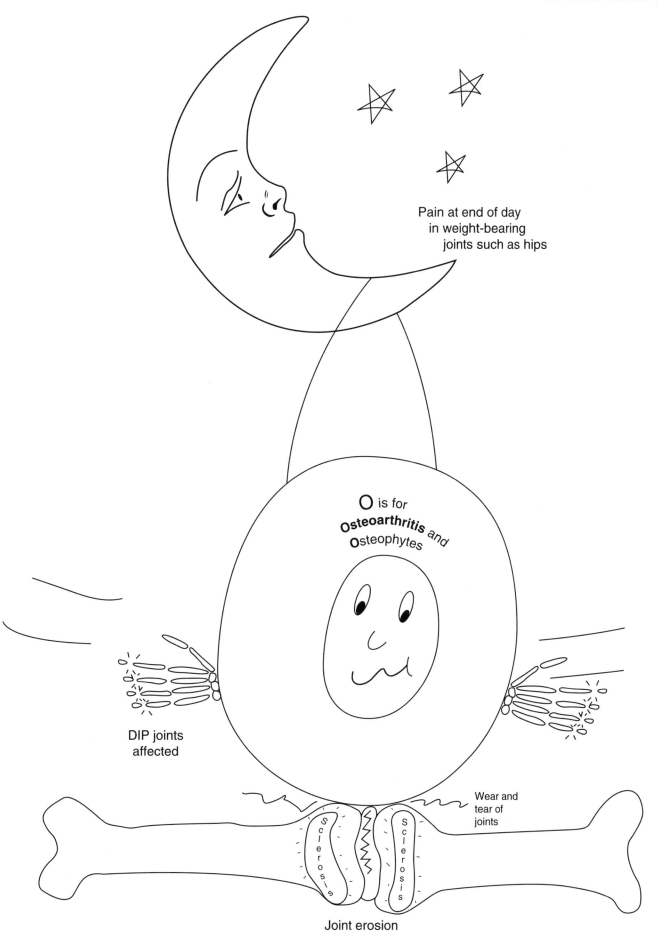

Pain at end of day
in weight-bearing
joints such as hips

O is for
Osteoarthritis and
Osteophytes

DIP joints
affected

Wear and
tear of
joints

Sclerosis

Sclerosis

Joint erosion

NOTES

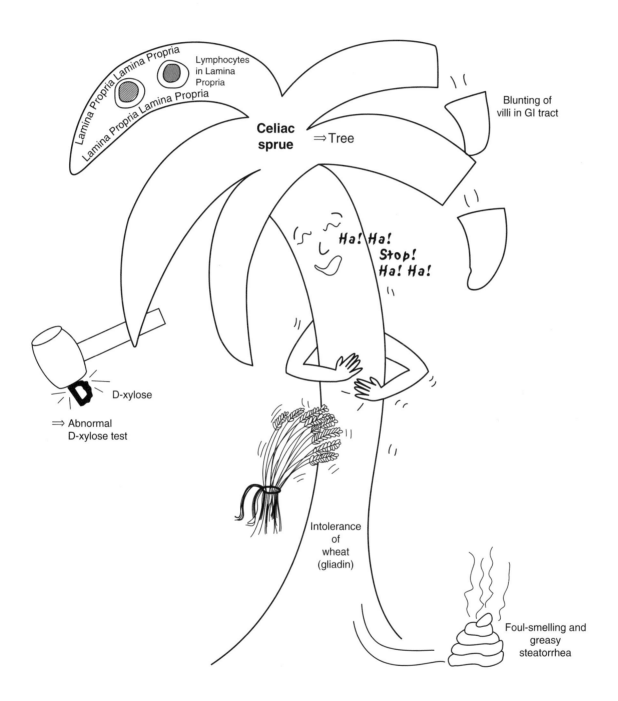

NOTES

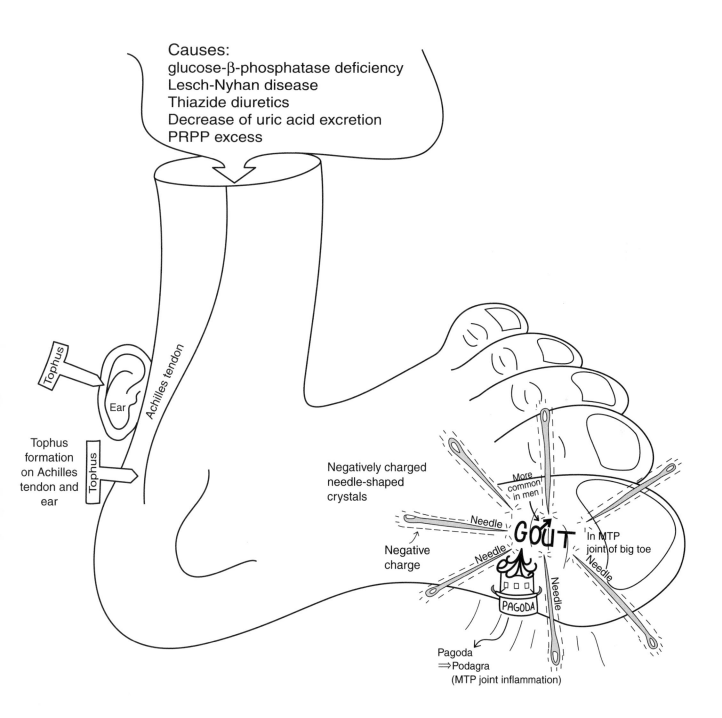

Causes:
glucose-β-phosphatase deficiency
Lesch-Nyhan disease
Thiazide diuretics
Decrease of uric acid excretion
PRPP excess

Tophus

Ear

Achilles tendon

Tophus
formation
on Achilles
tendon and
ear

Tophus

Negatively charged
needle-shaped
crystals

More
common
in men

Needle

Negative
charge

Needle

GOUT

In MTP
joint of big toe

Needle

Needle

PAGODA

Pagoda
⇒Podagra
(MTP joint inflammation)

NOTES

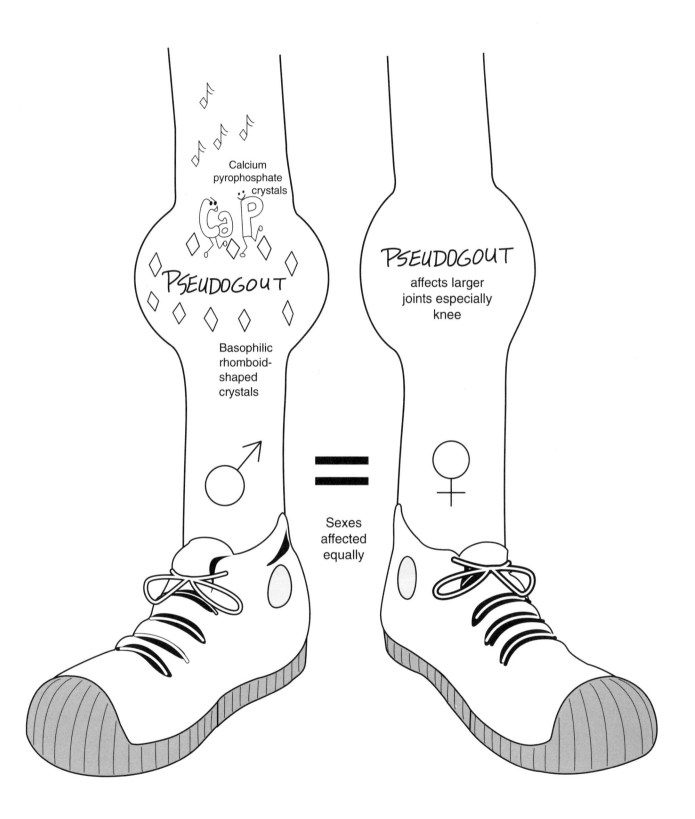

NOTES

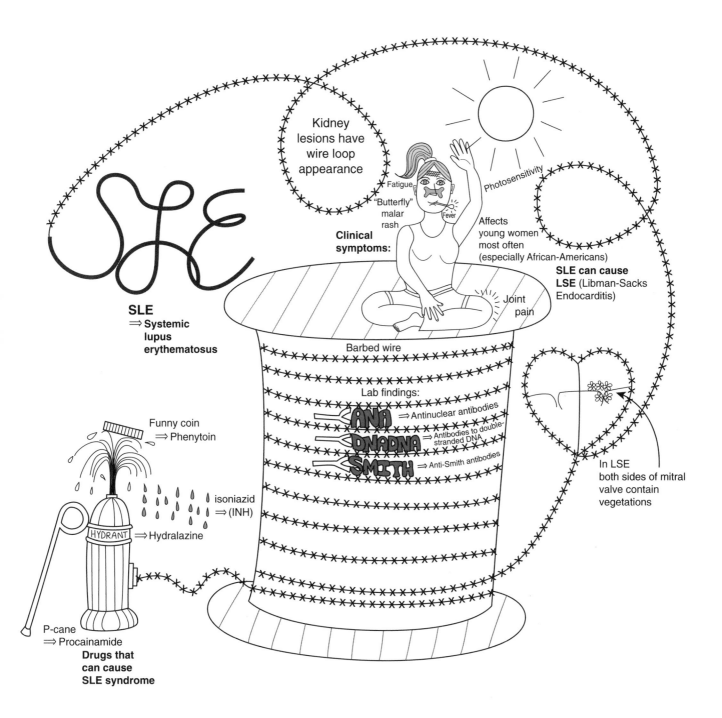

SLE
⇒ **Systemic lupus erythematosus**

Kidney lesions have wire loop appearance

Clinical symptoms:

Fatigue

"Butterfly" malar rash

Fever

Photosensitivity

Affects young women most often (especially African-Americans)

SLE can cause LSE (Libman-Sacks Endocarditis)

Joint pain

Barbed wire

Lab findings:

ANA ⇒ Antinuclear antibodies

DNADNA ⇒ Antibodies to double-stranded DNA

SMITH ⇒ Anti-Smith antibodies

In LSE both sides of mitral valve contain vegetations

Funny coin ⇒ Phenytoin

isoniazid ⇒ (INH)

HYDRANT ⇒ Hydralazine

P-cane ⇒ Procainamide
Drugs that can cause SLE syndrome

NOTES

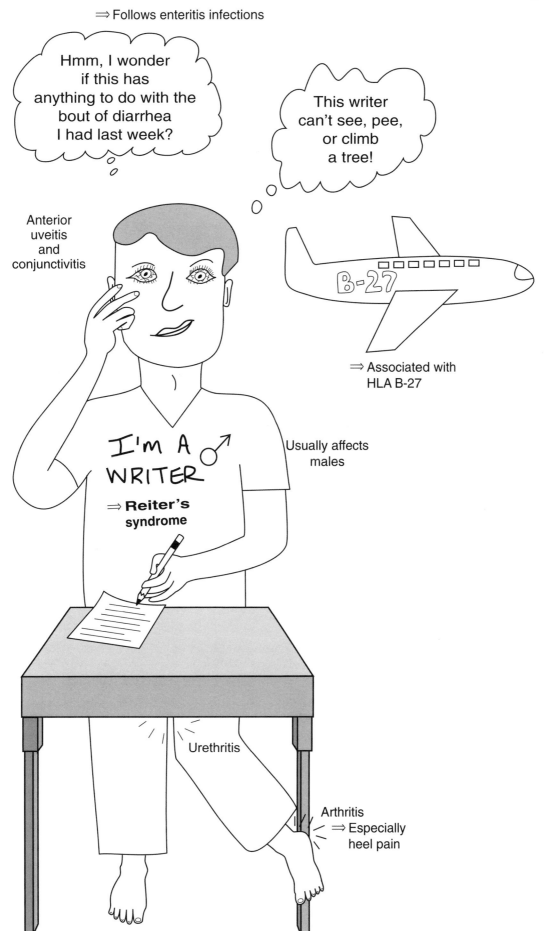

NOTES

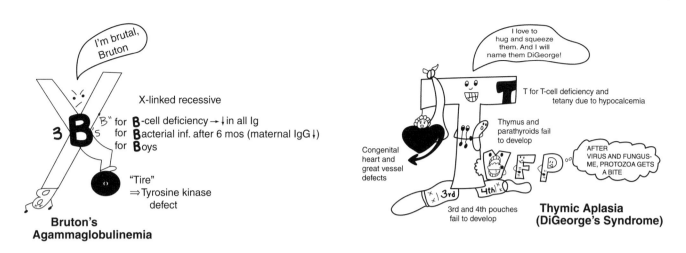

Bruton's Agammaglobulinemia

I'm brutal, Bruton

X-linked recessive

"B" for **B**-cell deficiency → ↓ in all Ig

"B" for **B**acterial inf. after 6 mos (maternal IgG↓)

"B" for **B**oys

"Tire" ⇒ Tyrosine kinase defect

I love to hug and squeeze them. And I will name them DiGeorge!

T for T-cell deficiency and tetany due to hypocalcemia

Thymus and parathyroids fail to develop

AFTER VIRUS AND FUNGUS-ME, PROTOZOA GETS A BITE

Congenital heart and great vessel defects

3rd and 4th pouches fail to develop

Thymic Aplasia (DiGeorge's Syndrome)

Chronic mucocutaneous candidiasis

"Chronic"

"CANADA"

CANDIDA

T-cell dysfunction specifically against *Candida albicans*

Recurrent infections with viral fungal protozoa

MHC II

Bacteria

Multiple causes:
- Failure to synthesize Class II MHC antigens
- Defective IL-2 receptors
- IL-2 adenosine deaminase deficiency

B- and T-cell deficiency

ADA

"SKID"
SCID—Severe combined immunodeficiency

IgA
IgA

Elevated IgA

Where's my Igm to get rid of this cap?

Capsular polysaccharides of bacteria

Eczema

Whiskey Alcohol

Recurrent pyogenic infection

Decreased platelets ⇒ In thrombocytopenia

B- and T-cell deficiency

Wiskott-Aldrich syndrome

CEREBELLAR ATAXIA

TAXI

"Cerebellar ataxia causes you to walk funny"

Spider angioma

Aarghh! A spider angioma!

IgA, T- and B-cell deficiency

Ataxia-telangiectasia

NOTES

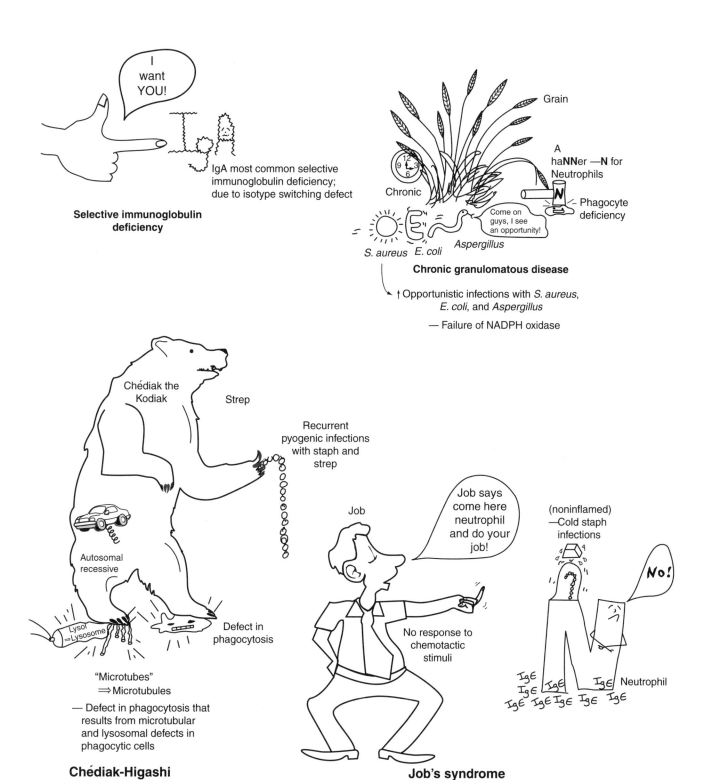

Selective immunoglobulin deficiency

IgA most common selective immunoglobulin deficiency; due to isotype switching defect

Chronic granulomatous disease

↑ Opportunistic infections with *S. aureus*, *E. coli*, and *Aspergillus*

— Failure of NADPH oxidase

Chédiak-Higashi disease

"Microtubes" ⇒ Microtubules

— Defect in phagocytosis that results from microtubular and lysosomal defects in phagocytic cells

Job's syndrome

NOTES

NOTES

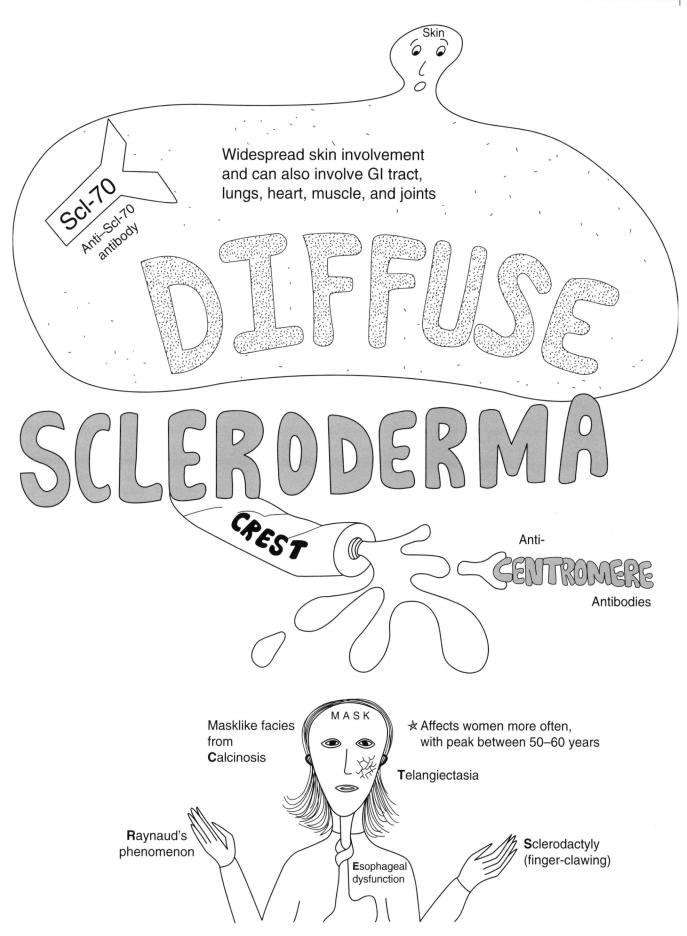

Skin

Scl-70
Anti–Scl-70 antibody

Widespread skin involvement and can also involve GI tract, lungs, heart, muscle, and joints

DIFFUSE

SCLERODERMA

CREST

Anti-
CENTROMERE
Antibodies

MASK

Masklike facies from **C**alcinosis

☆ Affects women more often, with peak between 50–60 years

Telangiectasia

Raynaud's phenomenon

Sclerodactyly (finger-clawing)

Esophageal dysfunction

NOTES

Sjögren's Sahara Desert

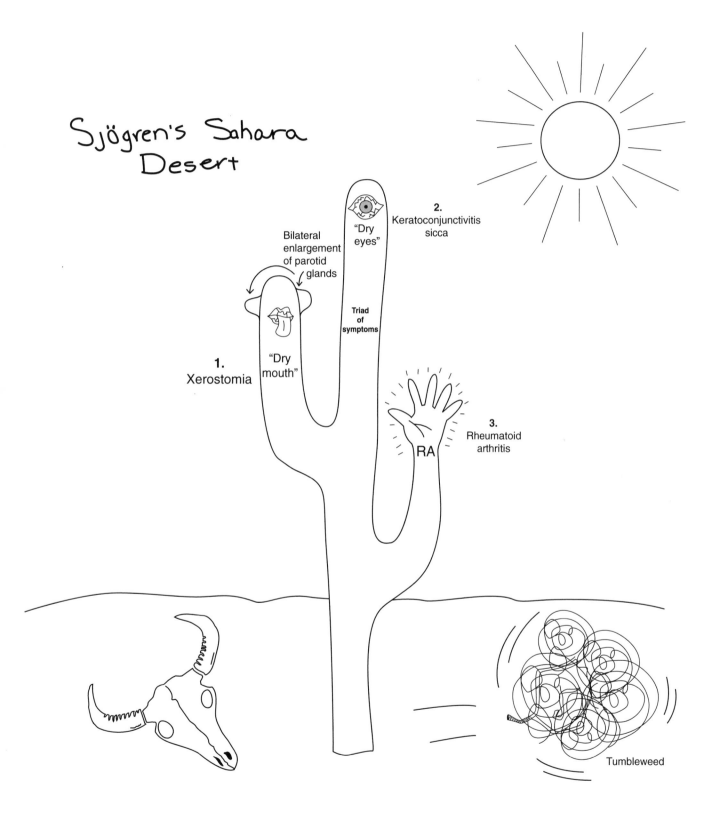

Bilateral enlargement of parotid glands

"Dry eyes"

2. Keratoconjunctivitis sicca

Triad of symptoms

1. Xerostomia

"Dry mouth"

RA

3. Rheumatoid arthritis

Tumbleweed

INDEX